Complementary & Alternative Therapies

An Implementation Guide to Integrative Health Care

Doris Milton, PhD, RN
Samuel Benjamin, MD

Health Forum, Inc.
An American Hospital Association Company
CHICAGO

AHA press

Printed in the United States of America—3/99

Cover design by Chip Butzko

Library of Congress Cataloging-in-Publication Data

Milton, Doris.
    Complementary and alternative therapies : an implementation guide to integrative health care / Doris Milton, Samuel Benjamin.
        p.   cm.
    Includes index.
    ISBN 1-55648-252-3 (pbk.)
    1. Alternative medicine.   2. Integrated delivery of health care.
I. Benjamin, Samuel (Samuel D.)   II. Title.
    [DNLM: 1. Alternative Medicine.   2. Delivery of Health Care,
Integrated—United States.   WB 890 M662c   1999]
    R733.M56   1999
    615.5—dc21
    DNLM/DLC
    for Library of Congress   98-45876
                                                   CIP

Item number: 067107

CONTENTS

ABOUT THE AUTHORS

Doris Milton, PhD, RN, is coeditor of *Alternative Therapies in Health and Medicine,* the largest interdisciplinary peer-reviewed journal in the field, and faculty at the University of Phoenix and Arizona State University. She has developed a continuing education program for nurses and other health care professionals and speaks frequently on alternative and complementary healing therapies and their integration into practice and education. She has published many articles in professional journals and authored several book chapters.

Dr. Milton's most recent position was as the founding director of research and education at The Arizona Center for Health and Medicine. She is an active member of Sigma Theta Tau, the international nursing honor society, and serves on the board of trustees of Nurse Healers-Professional Associates International Inc. She is an honorary member of Nurse Healers Therapeutic Touch Teachers Cooperative, a membership organization of approved Therapeutic Touch teachers. She has received awards for her teaching skills, mentorship, and contributions to research utilization in practice.

Dr. Milton is a graduate of St. Vincent's Medical Center School of Nursing in Staten Island, New York. She received her baccalaureate in nursing from Fairleigh Dickinson University and her master's and doctorate in nursing from New York University.

Samuel Benjamin, MD, is director of the University Center for Complementary and Alternative Medicine and associate professor, Clinical Pediatrics and Family Medicine, State University of New York at Stony Brook. Previously, he was the founding program director of the Arizona Center for Health and Medicine, an integrative group practice sponsored by Catholic Healthcare

West. He serves on the editorial board of *Alternative Therapies in Health and Medicine* and is a sought-after speaker on alternative and integrative medicine topics.

Dr. Benjamin received his medical degree from the University of Guadalajara; he studied herbal and indigenous medicine in Mexico. He completed a Fifth Pathway program at New York University Medical Center and was medical director of the first United States Urban Health Initiatives Program in the Bronx, New York. Dr. Benjamin has studied extensively in herbal and native healing therapies in Latin America and worked with the Tokyo Health Association to develop communitywide primary care programs.

Janet Kornblatt, JD, MPH, MA, received her law degree from Arizona State University and a master's in public health from the Columbia University School of Public Health. Her experience includes medical product liability, mass tort litigation, and medical malpractice defense. She has served as director, Urban Health Network Initiatives, Robert Wood Johnson Foundation and Montefiore Hospital, Bronx, New York, and as a program research analyst for the New York City Department of Health, Fraud and Abuse Unit.

This book is about integrative health care—the synthesis of complementary and alternative healing therapies with conventional health care. Today, people are less likely to accept unquestioningly the conventional interventions their health care practitioners may advise. They want to know all their options and be involved in the decisions that affect their health. As a result, consumers, health care professionals, and administrators are interested in keeping the best of conventional health care while integrating valid complementary and alternative approaches into that care.

Integrative health care requires much more than a business commitment to what might appear economically attractive in the marketplace. Organizations need to commit to and support a philosophy that accepts a new paradigm of practice. Integrative health care is more than merely adding in some "new" technologies, such as herbal preparations or acupuncture. Integration embraces patient self-empowerment and acknowledges the critical importance of leaving decision-making authority and many of the tools of healing within the patient's domain. In addition, integrative health care addresses disease prevention and the maintenance of one's own health with much more vigor than conventional care.

Experiencing alternative and complementary therapies allows many patients to recognize that there is something inside of themselves that has actually effected a change in health. This positive experience encourages them to seek similar experiences; for example, some people may feel empowered to use acupressure as a self-applied technology to relieve their pain. Those suffering from vascular headaches may choose to purchase the herb feverfew (a relatively inexpensive and potentially effective method of decreasing the frequency of vascular headaches) and avoid relying on conventional drugs.

If used as a "technology" alone, alternative and complementary therapies are just another value-added method that will have little impact on health care in the long term. While some institutions may see integrative health care only as a market differentiator, this perception would be quite erroneous. The public can and will spend dollars grudgingly on co-payments for managed care services or prescription plans, but willingly on care they perceive as helpful even if it is not reimbursed.

This book is designed to help all types of health care organizations—hospitals, health maintenance organizations, extended and ambulatory facilities, and solo or group practices—begin the integrative health care process. The material is designed to serve as a practical guide to address the challenges of this new paradigm.

Chapter 1 provides an overview of environmental factors influencing the development of integrative health care and the impact those factors may have in creating an integrative care program. Commonly used terms are defined, and the evolution of integrative care is summarized. The chapter ends with a discussion of the advantages of adopting an integrative health care model.

Chapter 2 describes a wide variety of the most commonly used complementary and alternative therapies or healing systems and is designed for those with little or no background in these areas. Information about desired qualifications of practitioners is provided when available.

Chapter 3 contains information for those who will be involved in the actual planning of an integrative project. Information is presented in a step-by-step format and includes strategies for forming a planning group, designing goals and objectives, selecting alternative therapies to integrate, and incorporating them into existing systems. Guidance is also provided on the important issues of credentialing and risk management, with particular emphasis on education and training needs. The importance of communication throughout the project is stressed.

Chapter 4 considers factors in the implementation phase of project development. The text highlights the importance of monitoring progress and describes how to develop an implementation monitoring plan. Strategies for dealing with opposition and the need for open communication are also discussed.

Chapter 5 lists the main tasks necessary to evaluate the outcomes of the integrative health care project. The components of the design, data collection, and data analysis steps are described and include suggestions for selecting outcomes measures, determining which data collection tools to use, and choosing an overall methodology. The importance of avoiding methodological errors is emphasized to ensure that results are accepted by the conventional health care community.

Chapter 6 provides a discussion of various issues that relate to the business side of integrative health care. The necessity of leadership commitment to the project's success is highlighted. Concerns regarding program structure, such as the organization's political climate, the physical environment for the program, and the availability of practitioners, are examined. The text provides budgeting and marketing strategies specific to integrative health care. In addition, detailed considerations for developing an alternative pharmacy—which is often separate from other elements of the care program—are described.

Chapter 7, written by Janet Kornblatt, JD, MPH, focuses on legal and regulatory issues involved in providing integrative health care in an independent practice or organizational setting. Strategies during all phases of the project are discussed, and helpful information is provided for consideration by the planning group, administration, and practitioners as they move health care into this new arena.

Appendix A contains resources and references: books, articles, organizations, and Web sites on integrative health care and selected alternative healing therapies and systems.

Appendix B provides brief overviews of integrative health care projects of various types. Some programs provide integrative care throughout an organization; others focus on a specific area or existing program. Some facilities are associated with health care systems, while others are stand-alone programs. No attempt was made to include all integrative efforts—there are too many to do so. However, this appendix provides the reader with a view of the wide array of possibilities that exist.

Integrative health care is one of the most exciting trends in health care today because it has the potential for improving quality of care and increasing practitioner satisfaction as well. People are entitled to the full array of valid health care options; integrative health care can help practitioners and organizations provide that level of care.

Overview of the Integrative Health Care Movement

Alternative and complementary healing therapies are being integrated into conventional health care to create a new paradigm called *integrative health care*. Environmental factors influencing its development and the many terms used to describe it are discussed in this chapter, as are its beginnings and the signs that it continues to evolve. The advantages of this health care model to patients, providers, organizations, and insurers are also described.

Environmental Factors Influencing Integrative Care

The integrative health care model is developing in many parts of the United States. Some consumers are interested in using alternative or complementary healing therapies exclusive of conventional health care, but most would prefer a blend of both approaches. And it is not just consumers who want all the options; health care professionals increasingly want to be able to provide them.

Integrative health care gives consumers and practitioners a model of care that is satisfying to both, with a palette of health care options. Providers are seeking alternative ways to return to what they originally wanted to be—healers. Spurred by various environmental factors, providers and consumers are increasingly choosing not to discard modern health care, but to complement it with alternative modalities that may be less expensive, as effective as conventional therapies, and opportunities for renewed and revitalized relationships between providers and patients. These environmental factors include rising health care costs, consumers' growing knowledge and concern about their health care choices, third-party payers' requirements, and both consumers' and providers' growing dissatisfaction with the limitations of allopathic health care.

Increasing Health Care Costs

The costs of health care in this country are projected to continue to rise due to the ongoing development of new and expensive technology and an aging population. People are living longer because of new technology and improved public health measures, better diet, and more exercise. There is a need to manage chronic disease and associated symptoms that affect the quality of life, not just its length.

Managed care has performed, at best, a containment function in relation to health care costs. It has limited the cost of care, but has not yet made any major inroads into actual cost reduction. Alternative and complementary therapies, which do not rely on invasive, high-tech procedures or synthetic medications, can often help manage symptoms and chronic disease at far lower cost than conventional methods. For example, acupuncture, massage, homeopathy, and/or changes in diet and exercise patterns may help people with osteoarthritis lessen or relieve pain without the use of expensive medications.

Dissatisfaction with the Present System

Many of the reasons for people's interest in changing the current health care system concern dissatisfaction with the present system and its limitations. With the highest per capita health care costs in the world, allopathic medicine in the United

States has done a lackluster job in showing that its strong emphasis on a "high-tech, low-touch" approach has significantly improved outcome criteria such as morbidity, mortality, or quality of life indices. People are troubled by the increased emphasis on equipment and technology and the lack of focus on people and their needs. Many believe there is an overemphasis on using antibiotics and invasive techniques, such as surgery and arteriograms, in situations in which there is little if any evidence of their effectiveness. Antibiotics are meeting increasing pathogen resistance caused by their frequent, and at times inappropriate, use. The media periodically express a fear of plagues sweeping the globe as a result of "supergerms."

The mainstream model of allopathic care is still an excellent choice for those with major trauma or for patients who need organ transplants, but it does not work as well for managing symptoms of chronic diseases or for many acute conditions such as colds, viruses, ear infections, sore throats, and bladder infections. Many consumers have already made a clear choice to use an alternative health care system to deal with chronic disease, an area in which the current allopathic system has not performed particularly well (Eisenberg et al. 1993; Landmark Healthcare 1998).

Increasing Interest in Health-Related Issues

Due to rising costs and dissatisfaction with conventional therapies, consumers are becoming better educated about a variety of factors that affect their health. It has become commonplace for news reports to include information about nutrition and food-related issues, and even in social settings, people discuss concerns such as food handling, nonlocal food supply, and the use of antibiotics and growth hormones in meat and poultry. People are interested not just in living longer, but also in living better, and there is a distinct movement back to more natural methods of eating and healing. To address these concerns, there is much emphasis in integrative health care on healthy eating, such as low-fat and vegetarian diets, organically-grown produce and meats, and free-range, hormone-free poultry. In addition, attention is being paid to such unconventional health-promoting activities as dance and music.

As they become more aware of alternative and complementary therapies, consumers are increasingly concerned about their lack of control over health care choices and the minimal input they have on the options available through their insurance programs. The costs of health care are increasing, yet the number of disability days lost from work is stable, or even increasing, in many corporations. Consumers are asked to pay more and more for their health insurance and copayments, yet the choices they have are decreasing. Authorization is needed in many plans for any appointment with a health care provider, and many care options that consumers want are uncovered. An increasing number of people use alternative therapies even though they are not covered by their insurance.

People are saying they want integrative care. They want only the treatment that is necessary, and they want all appropriate treatment options to be available to them. That interest crosses racial, ethnic, and gender lines and includes those with the highest incomes and educational levels. However, as the public and health care professionals ask more questions about integrative care, studies of integrative care and its outcomes cannot be performed unless there are places in which it is practiced. Also, current health care students need facilities in which to learn and practice integrative care.

The Medicolegal Environment

The public is frustrated with the current medicolegal environment as it interferes with the desired provider-patient relationship of shared decision making. People are aware that much of the current care they receive is provided solely to decrease physician and organization liability. Their concerns are heightened when the immediate reaction to a health care crisis is a flood of advertising from attorneys seeking those who feel they have been harmed. For example, the morning after news reports were released concerning the potential dangers in using Phen-Fen for weight loss, there were numerous ads on local television and radio stations asking people who had taken that drug combination to call attorneys if they had any questions about their rights. People want care that is more natural and less invasive, when possible—and they would prefer that all of this care, both conventional and alternative, be provided by a respected health care provider.

Integrative Health Care Terms

The variety of terms used in information related to integrative health care can sometimes be very confusing. Although they actually have different meanings, these terms are often used interchangeably. For example, those who integrate alternative therapies with conventional medicine tend to use the phrases "integrative" or "complementary" to describe their programs, even though some of the care provided or recommended is actually alternative care. This is because the former terms imply that conventional health care is not being discounted, but rather augmented.

Terminology is important because consumers need to know what type of care is provided; yet many proponents of integration hope to lessen the often emotionally reactive response of mainstream providers by using words such as *complementary*. This section defines and explains the most important and commonly used terms in integrative health care programs. Figure 1-1 provides a list of these terms with brief descriptions.

Alternative Healing Therapies

This term is used for therapies that can be substituted for more mainstream or conventional treatments or interventions. For example, men who have benign prostatic hyperplasia (BPH) can be treated with the herb saw palmetto (*Serenoa repens*) rather than the conventional prescribed medications. Saw palmetto improves the symptoms of BPH without the frequent side effects of conventional drugs.

Complementary Healing Therapies

Complementary is the term used for therapies that are used in addition to, rather than instead of, mainstream or conventional therapies. For example, people who have cancer often undergo conventional treatment with surgery, chemotherapy, and radiation. The use of such therapies as acupuncture, acupressure, guided imagery, Therapeutic Touch, nutritional supplements, herbal preparations, and homeopathic remedies can help people undergoing the necessary conventional treatment to improve their general health and manage the symptoms of cancer or side effects of treatment. So the use of these healing therapies in people with cancer is complementary rather than alternative.

Integrative Health Care

This is the term used for care that is a synthesis or blend of alternative, complementary, and mainstream or conventional

---

FIGURE 1-1. Definitions of Terms

Alternative Healing Therapies

   Modalities that can be used to substitute for a more mainstream or conventional treatment or intervention

Complementary Healing Therapies

   Modalities that are used in addition to, rather than instead of, a mainstream or conventional therapy

Healing Therapies

   Modalities, tools, treatments, or procedures used in any paradigm of health care

Healing Systems

   Paradigms or theoretical frameworks that define the perspective used for identification, diagnosis, and treatment of health problems

Holistic Health Care

   Care that focuses on the integration of body, mind, and spirit; a person is a whole human being and not just a sum of parts

Integrative Health Care

   Care that is a synthesis or blend of alternative, complementary, and mainstream or conventional care

---

care. There are few programs available to prepare health care professionals in integrative care. The Program in Integrative Medicine, under the leadership of Andrew Weil, MD, at the University of Arizona College of Medicine, is one of the most respected. The program accepts physicians who have completed a residency and who want to teach others interested in moving health care in the direction of integrative care.

Holistic Health Care

Many who use alternative and complementary therapies in their practice refer to their practices as "holistic." As discussed by Gordon (1996) in his book, *Manifesto for a New Medicine*, this term is currently most often used to describe a practice that is built on the integration of body, mind, and spirit; the person is viewed as a whole human being and not just a sum of parts. The term *holistic*, however, does not provide any information about whether or not the practitioner uses alternative, complementary, or conventional healing therapies, so its use can be confusing or misleading to the public and other practitioners.

Healing Systems and Healing Therapies

Some confusion occurs when different healing systems, such as Ayurveda, osteopathy, or Traditional Chinese Medicine, are discussed as if they were discrete, specific therapies. They are not modalities that can be taught as mere techniques, but rather are different systems of assessing people, making diagnoses, and providing treatment. Traditional Chinese Medicine, for example, is a system in which people's energy levels and imbalances are assessed and the skills of tongue and pulse diagnosis are used to determine the source of the problem and treatment plan. Moreover, many alternative or complementary healing therapies, although discussed as discrete entities (see chapter 2), are learned within a healing system such as Traditional Chinese Medicine. For example, acupuncture is not a therapy developed in isolation from a healing system; its use is based on theoretical premises from the Traditional Chinese Medicine system, and it is practiced within that framework.

Background of Complementary and Alternative Therapies

For many years, people have used alternative therapies without necessarily informing their physicians. However, this situation may be changing.

One of the major influences on the consideration of alternative therapies by the conventional medical community is the now classic study on nonconventional medicine in the United States published in *The New England Journal of Medicine* in 1993 (Eisenberg et al. 1993). That article reported the results of a study conducted by Eisenberg and colleagues at Harvard Medical School on the prevalence, costs, and patterns of use of alternative therapies in this country. The researchers limited their study to 16 therapies commonly used, but not taught widely in U.S. medical schools nor generally available in U.S. hospitals. They completed phone interviews with a national sample of 1,539 adults regarding any serious conditions and their use of conventional and nonconventional therapies. A third of the respondents reported using a nonconventional therapy in the previous year and a third of these saw providers for nonconventional therapies. The highest usage was reported by nonblack persons from 25 to 49 years of age who had relatively more education and higher incomes; therapies were used mostly for chronic conditions. Eighty-three percent also sought treatment for the same condition from a medical doctor, but 72 percent did not inform their physician that they had used or were using other therapies. Three-quarters of the amount spent for these therapies was paid out of pocket.

A recent survey published by Landmark Healthcare (1998) supports and extends these study findings. Telephone interviews were conducted using a random sample of households in this country; 1,500 interviews were completed. Participants were asked questions related to their attitudes, perceptions, usage, and actual behavior with regard to alternative health care. Forty-two percent of the sample had used some type of alternative care within the previous year; herbal therapy and chiropractic were the most prevalent types. Seventy-one percent thought that there would be a moderate or strong demand for alternative care in the future. Forty-five percent said that they would be willing to pay more in order to have access to alternative care, and 67 percent said that the availability of alternative care is an important consideration in their choice of a health plan. More people are informing their physician regarding their use of alternative care: 6 percent of this sample said that their physician knows they are seeking alternative care, and 45 percent say that their physician is very supportive of their doing so.

In addition, the findings of a national study concerning why people use alternative medicine were published in a recent issue of the *Journal of the American Medical Association (JAMA)* (Astin 1998). The majority of those using alternative therapies appear to be doing so not because they are dissatisfied with conventional medicine, but because the alternatives are more congruent with their values, beliefs, and philosophical orientations toward health and life.

In 1992, Congress established the Office of Alternative Medicine (OAM) within the National Institutes of Health (NIH); this office is responsible for establishing systems to evaluate the mechanisms and effects of varied alternative therapies. The OAM has funded many studies and research centers in the United States. One of the major projects undertaken by the OAM is an extensive report providing an overview of alternative therapies and their support, implications for future research, and an extensive reference list. A list of current research centers focusing on evaluating the use of varied alternative and complementary therapies is available through the NIH by phone or on its Web site (http://www.altmed.od.nih.gov/). The OAM has recently been elevated to Center status within the NIH.

The Movement toward Integration

Although slow, the progression toward integrative health care is growing. Demands from patients and providers have brought about change in several important areas, including practitioner education, available information, and insurance coverage.

Changes in Health Professional Education

At the present time, at least 30 medical schools in the United States include some content on alternative therapies in their curricula. Medical schools of the caliber of Harvard, Mount Sinai, Columbia, State University of New York at Stony Brook, and Georgetown offer such courses. Some medical schools integrate content in alternative medicine into required courses and others in electives. A detailed update of the courses available in medical schools can be found in the May 1998 issue of *Alternative Therapies in Health and Medicine* (Moore 1998). While there are no data as yet regarding integration of content and skills into the curricula of the formal educational programs in other health care disciplines, many colleges and schools offer such courses. For example, State University of New York at Stony Brook has a collaborative program in integrative health care that includes the programs in medicine, nursing, social work, occupational therapy, physical therapy, and dentistry, as well as in health sciences and technology management.

Continuing Education Programs

There has been a proliferation of continuing education programs related to integrative health care in general or focusing on specific alternative or complementary therapies or healing systems. For example, the journal *Alternative Therapies in Health and Medicine* holds an annual interdisciplinary conference focusing on various aspects of integrative health care. Harvard University sponsors an annual conference on spirituality and medicine, and Columbia University partners with other groups to sponsor ongoing continuing education programs in botanical medicine. Some programs are discipline-specific, such as the continuing education program on integrating alternative healing therapies into nursing practice and education sponsored by the University of Phoenix and *Alternative Therapies in Health and Medicine*. A sampling of conferences and contact information is provided in appendix A; readers will find that if they simply get their names on one or two lists, they will soon be receiving information from many sources about these educational opportunities.

Often, topics in the area of integrative health care or alternative and complementary therapies are also represented on the programs of conferences and meetings that focus mainly on conventional health care.

Availability of Information

There are many recently published books that represent the new wave of material available for individuals and organizations as they begin exploring this area. Some are written for health care professionals; examples of this type of book include *Manifesto for a New Medicine* (Gordon 1996), *Holistic Nursing: A Handbook for Practice* (Dossey et al. 1995), and the *American Holistic Nurses' Association Core Curriculum for Holistic Nursing Practice* (Dossey 1997). There are journals as well that reflect the increasing interest of health care professionals in this area. Representative are *Alternative Therapies in Health and Medicine* and the *Journal of Holistic Nursing*, while other journals, such as *Advances*, focus on a specific aspect of alternative healing.

There are an increasing number of books for the public as well. Titles such as *The Medical Advisor: The Complete Guide to Alternative and Conventional Treatments* (Time-Life Books 1996), and such magazines as *Natural Health* and *Self* are reflections of this trend. There are also publications that provide useful information to both health care professionals and the public; the newsletter *Self-Healing*, edited by Andrew Weil, MD, is such a resource. Appendix A provides a list of books, journal articles, and Web sites to help readers begin their research into the many facets of the field.

Of interest when examining trends is the fact that much information considered alternative ten years ago is now considered mainstream and is published in mainstream journals. For example, the work of Dean Ornish (Ornish et al. 1990; Gould et al. 1995) in examining the effects of a low-fat diet, exercise, and aspects of spirituality on coronary atherosclerosis is published in mainstream medical journals as well as alternative ones. The results of a survey published in *JAMA* showed a substantial variation between expert opinion and the opinion of readers as to the topics that *JAMA* should emphasize. Experts ranked alternative medicine sixty-eighth of 73 topics *JAMA* should publish, while readers ranked it seventh of 73. These findings were based on a survey mailed by *JAMA* in late 1996 and early 1997 to a stratified sample of 500 practicing physicians who are regular *JAMA* readers. The results of those surveys were compared with the results from the group of medical experts on whom *JAMA* typically relies (*Journal of the American Medical Association* 1998).

Insurance Coverage

In general, health care plan administrators express a great deal of interest in integrative health care, but they have several concerns about including alternative and complementary therapies as covered services. One of the most important is the credentialing process for therapy providers, especially for those who are not physicians or nurses. Insurers want to be as sure as they can that the therapies are practiced by legitimate providers, yet credentialing for many therapies is in the beginning stages or is nonexistent. Another stumbling block is that provision of most alternative and complementary therapies requires a system of billing codes, documentation, and claims processing separate from those for conventional procedures. Also, insurers are concerned that some therapies, such as massage, are attractive to many who have no specific medical need for them. Ways to ensure that those who need therapeutic massage are able to receive it, yet identify those for whom need cannot be determined, are necessary to keep such therapies from being misused as covered services. In general, insurers are concerned that covering these therapies may increase costs, yet they do not want to discourage those who could benefit from them. Plan administrators also know that many of their insureds are using these therapies without their physicians' knowledge, some of which have the potential for decreasing the effectiveness of conventional care or creating dangerous interactions with conventional care and medications. They do not want their insureds to be receiving care solely from an alternative provider, because that places plan participants at risk for a missed or late diagnosis by their physicians that could increase the costs of eventually needed services. At a minimum, plan administrators prefer health care providers who are knowledgeable regarding alternative and complementary therapies and who can plan and manage patient care problems using an integrative approach.

Although alternative and complementary therapies are only in the beginning phases of being considered routinely covered services, some health insurance plans do include selected therapies, at least as a rider to a conventional policy. In addition, some stand-alone discounted networks are available in many parts of the country. For example, the Complementary Care Company, based in Maryland, provides individual, student, and family members with access to alternative health care providers who have agreed to a fixed discounted fee or a specific percentage discount to plan members. More than 50 alternative health care services are available, as is assistance in selecting the appropriate provider. Many similar programs include overall health promotion counseling and educational programs, as well as networks of alternative providers. Networks of providers are becoming increasingly popular because of the public's perception that someone has screened provider qualifications prior to their inclusion in the network. However, screening methods are as varied as the networks. American Specialty Health Plans in California, the nation's largest subcontractor of alternative and complementary health care providers, addresses both credentialing and quality of care issues. The plan currently has approximately three million insureds.

Insurers that have shown an interest in integrative health care systems include conventional indemnity plans, preferred provider organizations, individual practice associations, and managed care plans, and this trend seems likely to continue. For example, a study completed in 1997 by the Landmark Foundation, a chiropractic-supported foundation based in Sacramento, found that over 100 managed care companies (58 percent) surveyed in 14 states planned to cover at least some complementary and alternative medicines within the following 24 months. The Oxford Health Plan in the northeastern United States began to cover complementary and alternative medicine in 1996, developing its own standards for credentialing.

Advantages of Integrating Alternative and Complementary Therapies

The willingness to satisfy the demands of consumers, practitioners, and third-party payers will greatly determine health care organizations' ability to survive in the coming years.

Offering integrative health care at reasonable costs may be one of the most important ways of addressing these demands.

Meeting Consumer Needs

There are many advantages to health care systems, health maintenance organizations, and group practices in integrating alternative therapies into their conventional programs. It can be seen by consumers as a response to their wish for more responsibility and control over the health care they receive. People are seeking care from practitioners and organizations providing the most options from which they can choose. Their preference is "one-stop shopping" for health care; that is, they want to be able to select from an array of conventional and alternative care therapies without having to go to several locations. Moreover, many providers are hopeful that allowing people a greater array of health care choices will, in turn, increase the likelihood of their assuming more responsibility for lifestyle choices that improve their health. In addition, many consumers today are committed to improving the larger environment and taking a role in the health of the communities in which they live, and integration of alternative therapies can fit into that larger picture.

Market Differentiation

Offering integrative health care helps to differentiate an organization or group practice in the marketplace. Offering this type of care presents an image of being on the "cutting edge" and committed to providing the types of care that consumers want. Development of integrative health care programs also facilitates a different type of involvement with the community than most organizations have. Including community leaders and members in the process of selecting which alternative therapies will be integrated can, in turn, benefit the organization. For example, health care facilities in many areas of the United States serve Native Americans, yet the health care views and practices of these populations have been ignored. Studying and incorporating them could benefit the whole community and make the organization more attractive to its special populations.

Potential Cost Savings

Another major concern of those who receive or pay for health care is the increasing cost of services and technology. Overall, integrative health care involves fewer diagnostic tests and less expensive treatment modalities in the long term. Many alternative or complementary therapies are much less expensive than conventional care and, because of their emphasis on patient empowerment and responsibility for health, less provider time is needed.

Increased Provider Satisfaction

Many health care practitioners today complain of their decreasing satisfaction with their work because so much of what they do is not individualized—care is provided in a "cookie cutter" manner according to a standardized protocol from which little deviation is permitted. Integrating many of the alternative therapies into standardized care allows practitioners to provide the best possible care tailored to the individual. Within current time restraints for providing care, integrative health care allows practitioners to offer a wide array of options, both allopathic and alternative. In integrative health care, the protocols for common patient problems or conditions is a menu of options, rather than a prescribed list of diagnostic tests and treatments. Integrating these care options allows practitioners to reconnect with patients and treat them as individuals by listening to them and developing plans of care specific to their needs. This type of care is more satisfying to both providers and patients.

Conclusion

The integration of alternative and complementary healing therapies into conventional health care is of increasing interest to both the public and health care professionals. Information regarding these therapies is proliferating, and health care systems need to consider which therapies they might begin integrating into care—or whether they want to integrate these therapies at all. Given their advantages to health care systems, practitioners, insurers, and consumers, it is important to become familiar with some of the more commonly used alternative and complementary healing therapies. The next chapter provides the reader with an overview of some of these therapies and examples of their use.

References Cited

Astin, J. A. 1998. Why patients use alternative medicine: Results of a national study. *Journal of the American Medical Association* 279 (19): 1548–53.

Dossey, B. M. 1997. *American Holistic Nurses' Association Core Curriculum for Holistic Nursing Practice*. Gaithersburg, MD: Aspen.

Dossey, B. M., L. Keegan, C. E. Guzzetta, and L. G. Kolkmeier. 1995. *Holistic Nursing: A Handbook for Practice*. 2d ed. Gaithersburg, MD: Aspen.

Eisenberg, D. M., et al. 1993. Unconventional medicine in the United States. *The New England Journal of Medicine* 328 (4): 246–51.

Gordon, J. 1996. *Manifesto for a New Medicine: Your Guide to Healing Partnerships and the Wise Use of Alternative Therapies*. Reading, MA: Addison Wesley.

Gould, K. L., D. Ornish, L. Scherwitz, S. Brown, R. P. Edens, M. J. Hess, N. Mullani, F. Dobbs, W. T. Armstrong, T. Merritt, T. Ports, S. Sparier, and J. Billings. 1995. Changes in myocardial perfusion abnormalities by positron emission tomography after long-term, intense risk-factor modification. *Journal of the American Medical Association* 274 (11): 894–901.

Journal of the American Medical Association. 1998. Results of a reader survey. *Journal of the American Medical Association* 280: 296–98.

Landmark Healthcare & Interactive Solutions. 1998. *The Landmark Report on Public Perceptions of Alternative Care.* Sacramento, CA: Landmark.

Moore, N. 1998. A review of alternative medicine courses taught at US medical schools. *Alternative Therapies in Health and Medicine* 4 (3): 90–99, 100–101.

Ornish, D., S. E. Brown, L. W. Scherwitz, J. H. Billings, W. T. Armstrong, T. A. Ports, S. M. McLanahan, R. L. Kirkeeide, R. J. Brand, and K. L. Gould. 1990. Can lifestyle changes reverse coronary heart disease? *The Lancet* 336: 129–33.

Time-Life Books. 1996. *The Medical Advisor: The Complete Guide to Alternative and Conventional Treatments.* New York: Time-Life Books.

Overview of Complementary and Alternative Healing Therapies

This chapter provides an overview of alternative healing systems and commonly used alternative and complementary therapies. The focus is on those therapies most frequently used by professional providers and considered by many to be appropriate for integration into conventional care. This information will be helpful for those with little or no background in the field. Whenever applicable, the qualifications for practitioners of these therapies are provided. Those who wish to learn more about a specific therapy or the credentialing or training organizations mentioned should refer to the selected reference list in appendix A at the end of this book.

The therapies and healing systems are presented in alphabetical order. Readers will note that the word *energy* or its equivalents are used in the descriptions of many of these therapies. Whether or not one believes that energy actually moves, becomes imbalanced, or changes, these ideas may be viewed figuratively.

Integrative health care supports the notion that instead of an alternative science there is one science that pervades the universe and that many alternative and complementary therapies may represent areas of life sciences that we simply have not explored yet. It is important to point out that in many cases there are insufficient data to be sure of what works and what does not; however, this is hardly different from allopathic care, in which much treatment is based on theoretical supposition.

Acupressure

Acupressure involves using pressure with the fingers on the same points in which needles are used in acupuncture. It is thought to change the energy flow through the body, leading to symptom relief or an improvement in the sense of well-being. Acupressure is effective for many of the same symptoms as acupuncture, but can take longer to provide symptom relief.

One commonly used acupressure treatment has been shown to be effective in helping to relieve headaches. The Large Intestine 4, the fleshy portion (the part between the thumb and index finger) of the hand, is squeezed between the thumb and index finger of the opposite hand for one to two minutes. This treatment should not be used during pregnancy. Another commonly used acupressure point, called Pericardium 6, can be helpful for people who suffer from nausea. The thumb of one hand is placed firmly on the center of the opposite inner wrist, two fingers down from where the wrist creases, for one to two minutes. The pressure is then repeated on the other arm and reapplied to both as often as needed.

No special training is needed for acupressure, and patients can use acupressure for self-healing or to help others. There are many books available that demonstrate the common acupressure points using pictures and easy-to-follow directions.

Acupuncture

One of the more commonly used alternative therapies, acupuncture involves the use of needles to manipulate the body's network of energy pathways (called *meridians*) to activate the body's energy, or *qi*. Meridians can be thought of as highways along which the vital energy of the body flows; these meridians are not aligned with nerve structures or blood vessels. Small needles are inserted at appropriate points in various combinations and patterns and then left in place for varying amounts of time, usually from 8 to 20 minutes. Acupuncture needles are solid and hairlike, causing only momentary discomfort, if any, when they are inserted. Heat can be applied to the ends of the needles by burning an herbal substance called *moxa*. Alternatively, low-level electrical stimulation can be used to increase stimulation of the acupuncture points.

Acupuncture can be useful in managing acute or chronic pain. Although the mechanism of action of acupuncture is unclear, it is thought to work by releasing neurotransmitters, such as endorphins. Its ability to provide long-lasting pain relief, however, cannot be explained by that mechanism. Acupuncture is also beneficial for such symptoms as nausea and vomiting, constipation and diarrhea, fatigue or general malaise, and back discomfort. The National Institutes of Health released a consensus statement in 1997 that said there is "clear evidence that needle acupuncture treatment is effective for postoperative and chemotherapy nausea and vomiting, nausea of pregnancy, and postoperative dental pain." The 12-member expert panel also concluded that there are a number of other pain-related conditions for which acupuncture "may be effective as an adjunct therapy, an acceptable alternative, or as part of a comprehensive treatment program, but for which there is less convincing scientific data." These conditions include headache, lower back pain, addiction, stroke rehabilitation, menstrual cramps, tennis elbow, fibromyalgia, carpal tunnel syndrome, and asthma (Villaire 1998).

In many states, acupuncturists are licensed or must meet training or registration requirements for practice. In other states, acupuncture is included in the scope of practice, so the medical practice of this therapy is not regulated or restricted. Physicians who practice acupuncture may be certified by the American Academy of Medical Acupuncture (AAMA), which includes a proficiency examination and requirements for formal training and clinical experience as components of its certification process. Membership in the AAMA has become the standard for physician credentialing in acupuncture (Helms 1998). Many states regulate the practice of acupuncture by providers other than physicians, although the requirements vary widely. The most recognized group to credential these nonphysician providers is the National Commission for the Certification of

Acupuncturists, which has developed a national examination for applicants. One of the major concerns for consumers is to be sure that sterile, disposable needles are used to prevent the spread of bloodborne disease.

Ayurvedic Medicine

This is an ancient healing system that uses the quality of the pulse to assess the balance of the *doshas*, or three core principles termed *kapha*, *pitta*, and *vata*. Imbalance in the doshas is thought to create symptoms and disease. Treatment is designed to correct the imbalances and consists of herbs, nutrition, and oil massages. The patient's entire lifestyle, including time of day for waking and sleeping, eating, massage, and other activities, is considered very important in this healing system. Ayurvedic practitioners also use a variety of mind-body techniques, such as meditation and yoga.

There is no nationally recognized program to prepare or credential ayurvedic practitioners.

Herbal Remedies

Herbal preparations are used to balance the body's energies and treat specific illnesses. Several herbs can be helpful in relieving a variety of common symptoms. Chamomile or ginger, frequently used as teas, can have a calming effect for gastritis or irritable bowel. Chamomile can also be helpful for stress and anxiety. Some mushrooms, especially shiitake or maitake, have been found to enhance immune system function. Either valerian or kava kava can be used for anxiety or insomnia. Garlic is helpful for those with infections; many preparations are concentrated and do not have the characteristic garlic odor. Garlic has many benefits: it is a natural antibiotic and affects the cardiovascular system by lowering blood cholesterol and blood pressure in many people. Ginger and gugulipid can also be helpful in lowering blood cholesterol, as well as in improving the ratio of high-density to low-density lipoproteins.

Herbal preparations can interact with prescription medicines, so it is important to check potential drug-herb interactions. For example, St. John's wort, an herb commonly used for depression, is thought to work in a fashion similar to widely used prescription antidepressants, so people should not take both simultaneously. Ginger is recommended for nausea and other gastrointestinal upsets, but it can increase the bleeding risk in people who are taking warfarin or aspirin. Some herbs, such as black cohosh, work in a manner similar to estrogen and should not be used during pregnancy.

Herbs do not require prescriptions, although they are the basis for many prescription drugs. Herbal preparations are not regulated, so consumers need to obtain them from a reputable source. Those sold as standardized extracts are more likely to contain the accurate amount of active component of the herb as stated on the label, and less likely to contain inactive plant parts or pesticides, than do products that are not standardized. The only reassurance that consumers have at this time that they are obtaining a high-quality product is that many manufacturers have stringent quality-control procedures, including random audits and independent laboratory testing of products.

There is no standard credentialing process for practitioners who integrate the use of herbal preparations with other therapies. However, those who have been educated in healing systems, such as naturopathic medicine or Traditional Chinese or Oriental Medicine, usually have had considerable instruction regarding the use of herbs.

Homeopathy

Homeopathy is a system of healing developed in the late eighteenth century based on the "law of similars." This principle states that a much diluted preparation of a substance that can cause symptoms in a healthy person can cure those same symptoms in a sick person. Homeopathic medicines, called *remedies*, are made from naturally occurring plant, animal, and mineral substances, some of which (such as arsenic) are poisonous. Homeopathic preparations are so diluted, however, that it is impossible to poison a patient; in fact, most remedies have no detectable amount of the original substance. Homeopathic preparations are available in different dilutions or potencies; the more dilute the preparation, the more potent it is thought to be.

People receiving treatment from a practitioner known as a *constitutional homeopath* receive remedies that are individualized: two or more people with the same diagnosis may be given different remedies, depending on the specific symptoms of each person. In contrast, some homeopathic practitioners treat acute symptoms with over-the-counter preparations that are combinations of the most commonly used homeopathic remedies for a specific symptom.

Homeopathic remedies are usually available in tablet form; the tablets are very small and are usually used sublingually. Some remedies are also available as liquids or tinctures, and there is even a homeopathic cream used for muscle sprains, strains, and injuries. The dosage frequency varies with the type of problem and the potency of the remedy. Practitioners frequently advise those using homeopathic remedies to avoid coffee (even decaffeinated) and mint because they are believed to hamper the effectiveness of remedies. Relief of symptoms can occur in a few minutes to a few days. Because homeopathy is thought to work by stimulating the body's natural healing abilities, people can stop taking the remedy once symptoms have begun to decrease.

The manufacture of homeopathic preparations is regulated by the Food and Drug Administration (FDA), so these remedies are safe to purchase over the counter. The educational preparation of constitutional or classic homeopaths is lengthy, but laypeople can "experiment" with remedies for acute conditions by following the information available on packaging or by using references available for lay use, such as the guide written by Cummings and Ullman (1991). Programs and materials are also available through the National Center for Homeopathy. Common homeopathic preparations for many symptoms are often available in health food stores, and directions for taking the remedies are on the label or in booklets provided by the manufacturer. If over-the-counter homeopathic remedies are not helpful, people may seek out an expert homeopathic practitioner for symptom relief.

There is no standardized educational program for homeopathy, but several reputable programs exist. The Hahnemann

College of Homeopathy offers a four-year curriculum that prepares health professionals and the public who wish to practice homeopathy. Physicians who practice homeopathy can be certified through the American Institute of Homeopathy. Physicians who practice homeopathy in Arizona, Connecticut, and Nevada must be licensed by both the allopathic board and the board of homeopathic examiners in those states.

Imagery

Imagery is the use of all the senses to encourage changes in attitudes, behavior, and physiological reactions. Numerous studies have supported the positive effects that imagery, either alone or in combination with other alternative therapies, can have on outcomes for people with diseases such as cancer when integrated with conventional care. For example, a study conducted by Frank (1985) found that guided visual imagery, when used in combination with music therapy, could have a positive effect on anxiety and perceived degree of vomiting in people with cancer who are undergoing chemotherapy.

Imagery can be divided into several types. Visualization is a specific form of imagery, allowing a person to see something with the mind's eye. Practitioners may use a form of imagery called interactive guided imagery, which allows a person to communicate with a symptom, to help identify ways of relieving distress (Rossman 1987). Imagery can also be used to treat depression, anxiety, and stress by helping people to understand the connections between stressful circumstances and physical symptoms and showing them ways to release unconscious blocks to relief and improvement. Imagery does not have to be complicated to be effective. People can be encouraged to use a relaxation technique and then create any image that they find helps to reduce their stress or deal with a particular symptom. Sample scripts that can be used for specific concerns can be found in Rossman (1987) and Dossey et al. (1995).

There is no standardized national educational or licensing requirement for the practice of imagery, but there are several established programs held in high regard. Programs in guided imagery are available, both as classes and on a home-study basis, through the Academy for Guided Imagery. A special version of that program, sponsored by the American Holistic Nurses' Association, is designed for nurses. Also, there are many reputable training programs in imagery; information about those programs is readily available in scholarly journals.

Music Therapy

Music therapy is the use of sound to promote relaxation and reduce stress and pain. Music is an inexpensive therapy and, because of its familiarity, can be less threatening when people are beginning to explore alternative therapies. Inexpensive audiocassettes or compact discs can be used; music seems to work better if people select the type of music they prefer. In her study examining the use of music for cancer-related pain, Beck (1991) found that the most popular types of music chosen for relaxation were easy listening, country and western, and classical. Many practitioners and others in care settings may be willing to donate tapes or compact discs.

There is no standardized preparation for music therapy. Names of qualified music therapists can be obtained from the National Association of Music Therapists.

Naturopathic Medicine

Naturopathy is a healing system that uses natural treatments, rather than those that are synthetic or invasive, whenever possible to remove or reduce the cause of symptoms or disease. Therapies commonly used by naturopathic physicians include nutrition and diet, acupuncture, herbal preparations, and exercise.

Naturopathic physicians receive preparation in naturopathic medical schools; the curriculum is four years in length. Graduates, who use the initials N.D. to denote their preparation, are licensed to practice in some states. The most well-known naturopathic medical school is Bastyr in the state of Washington, one of the sites conducting research sponsored by the Office of Alternative Medicine (a division of the NIH). The focus of this program is the study of the use of alternative therapies for those persons with HIV/AIDS.

Nutrition and Nutritional Supplements

Nutrition and nutritional supplements include the use of foods, vitamins, and other nutritional materials to promote health and to treat some disease symptoms or effects. Most people know that they need to take vitamins or nutritional supplements on a regular basis, but many are not sure which are most effective or what dosage is needed. There are several reputable sources of advice; for example, the recommendations of experts such as Weil (1995) and Murray (1996) can be used. More information becomes available on an almost daily basis about the role of foods and selected nutrients in the prevention of diseases or the enhancement of immune system functioning.

One common nutritional supplement that has implications for those with cardiovascular problems is coenzyme Q10, an essential component of cellular physiology that is thought to play a major role in cellular energy production and acts as an antioxidant. This naturally occurring substance, when used as a supplement, helps to decrease symptoms in those with mild to moderate congestive heart failure. Also, many practitioners think that coenzyme Q10 plays an important role in cancer prevention and treatment and may help to reduce cardiotoxicity associated with some chemotherapeutic agents.

Improvement in many people with osteoarthritis can be seen when the nutritional supplement glucosamine sulfate is used. It is very well tolerated and can help relieve discomfort or pain through the regeneration of cartilage.

Of great interest is the program developed by Ornish for people with coronary disease. The program has a 10-percent fat, vegetarian diet as its cornerstone; moderate exercise, yoga, spirituality, and participation in support groups are included as well. Ornish and his colleagues have published the outcomes of actual reversal of the process of atherosclerosis in conventional medical journals (Gould et al. 1995; Ornish et al. 1990). Programs such as this one demonstrate the powerful effects of nutrition and exercise on serious clinical conditions.

There is no standardized educational program in the area of nutrition and nutritional supplements. In fact, many health care professionals who have been educated in mainstream programs are not familiar with nutritional supplements and their uses. Practitioners who have naturopathic medical preparation usually receive extensive instruction in this area.

Osteopathy and Osteopathic Manipulation Techniques

Osteopathic manipulation techniques are used in osteopathy, a system of medicine based on sensing the health of the body as an integrated unit, acknowledging the interrelationship of structure and function, and using the body's own self-healing mechanisms. Osteopathic physicians sense pulsations or restricted motion in the body and use gentle manipulative techniques to treat a wide variety of abnormalities and help the body return to normal or optimal functioning. Osteopathic manipulation can be effective in reducing symptoms for people who have pain of any kind, respiratory difficulties, muscle spasms, gastrointestinal problems, or stress; many use osteopathic manipulation to maintain their health as well.

Not all osteopathic physicians specialize in manipulative techniques; osteopathy is a holistic system that also includes instruction in proper posture, body mechanics, and exercise, as well as consideration of psychological influences, lifestyle choices, and nutrition. Providers who have continued their training in manipulation beyond the basic educational preparation become Doctors of Osteopathy.

Reflexology

Reflexology is a form of massage applied to the foot or hand. It is based on the premise that any discomfort or pain in a specific area of the foot or hand indicates a disease or disorder in a corresponding body part. Pressure on the correct area of the foot or hand is thought to release the blockage in that area and allow energy to flow freely through that related part of the body.

Although there are lengthy programs in reflexology, some of the basics can be learned easily. Also, color-coded charts are available that show the locations of corresponding foot or hand sites. Laypeople can use these charts to locate the appropriate point on the foot to massage in order to relieve symptoms. There is no national credentialing standard for reflexology, but the International Institute of Reflexology sponsors highly regarded certification programs.

Spirituality and Prayer

Spirituality and prayer are used to assist people in finding an inner sense of something greater than the individual self or in perceiving meaning that transcends the immediate circumstances. Spirituality is a sense of meaning and purpose in life or a belief in a higher power or source of energy without any limits. It involves a person's core or soul and the need to reach out beyond the self. Prayer can be the outward, concrete expression of such feelings, although not all people meet their spiritual needs through prayer or an organized form of religion.

When people are faced with a life-threatening diagnosis or need to deal with symptoms that will change their lifestyle, spiritual interventions can be most helpful. Although there are many ways in which health care practitioners can help people at this time (Bauer and Barron 1993), many traditional caring behaviors can be supportive of people's spiritual needs. If patients are religious, it can be very powerful for providers to take a few minutes to pray with them, not only for a positive outcome, but also for strength during a time of crisis.

Support Groups

Support groups are gatherings of people with common conditions or issues; members are encouraged to discuss their feelings, including fears, and their experiences with disease or its treatment. Other therapies can be included as part of the session, but the main benefits of participation seem to be that, through frequent meetings, group members grow to care for each other, understand each other's feelings and problems, and provide support during treatment and recovery. For example, the results of a now classic study (Spiegel et al. 1989) showed that women with breast cancer who had taken part in support groups lived an average of 18 months longer than those who did not. Support groups seem especially helpful not only for those with cancer, but also for those trying to make lifestyle changes, such as with diet and exercise, or those in the rehabilitation phase of treatment (such as a substance abuse program).

Therapeutic Touch

Therapeutic Touch (TT) involves using the palms of the hands, held two to three inches away from a person's body, to sense energy imbalances, correct those imbalances, and help the energy flow smoothly throughout the body. Therapeutic Touch is based on the theory that a healthy person has no imbalances; energy is evenly distributed throughout the body and flows freely and smoothly with no blocks to its movement. It is believed that energy does not really stop where the physical body does, so that energy can be felt from several inches away. The energy is supposed to feel the same all over, front and back, head to foot, on both sides of the body. When a TT practitioner senses a difference in one part of the body, it may be felt as a difference in temperature (not connected with actual skin temperature), a difference in volume (one area feels heavier or lighter), or a difference in "staticky" feeling (as in static electricity). Any of the differences can be felt in various areas of the body.

Therapeutic Touch can be helpful in treating conditions of acute pain (for example, headache or pain after an operation) or chronic pain (as with arthritis). It can be helpful as well in reducing stress. People report being less anxious or tense and much calmer after treatment; many say it feels as if they have had a good night's sleep. One of its most beneficial effects is its impact on wound healing. A series of research studies have shown that TT accelerates the rate of wound healing (Wirth et al. 1993; Wirth et al. 1994; Wirth et al. 1996), which can be very beneficial to those recovering from surgical or other invasive procedures, such as the insertion of ports for medication administration. Also, TT may help to relieve the discomfort of breathing problems associated with colds or sore throats.

An entire TT treatment takes 10 to 15 minutes. As with many other complementary therapies, TT rarely has side effects and does not interfere with any medication or other treatment. Anyone, even those without a health care background, can learn the basics of Therapeutic Touch in a one- or two-day workshop from a reputable teacher. There are no certification programs in Therapeutic Touch, but nurses and other health care professionals who are expert Therapeutic Touch teachers are approved by the Nurse Healers–Professional Associates International, Inc.

Traditional Chinese Medicine

Traditional Chinese Medicine is an ancient healing system that uses assessment of the tongue and the quality of the pulse to determine imbalances in the flow of energy through a person's body. Treatment of energy balances uses combinations of herbs, acupuncture, and nutrition.

There is no national standardized program to train practitioners in this healing system, but there are many reputable oriental medicine programs in various parts of the country.

The Trager Approach

The Trager approach is a form of bodywork that uses light, rhythmic rocking and shaking movements that loosen joints, ease movement, and release chronic tension patterns. Practitioners use their hands to influence deep-seated patterns in the recipient's mind and interrupt their projection into body tissues. The Trager method is especially beneficial to those with chronic diseases that have associated muscle patterns that cause discomfort; for example, arthritis, fibromyalgia, and multiple sclerosis.

Practitioners of Trager are certified through the Trager Institute.

Conclusion

The selection of alternative and complementary therapies described in this chapter is not meant to be inclusive; it is intended to provide an overview of the variety of therapies available for various uses. Readers are encouraged to use this information as a starting point for further research on these and additional therapies that may apply to specific areas of interest in conventional treatment.

References Cited

Bauer, T., and C. R. Barron. 1993. Nursing interventions for spiritual care. *Journal of Holistic Nursing* 13 (3): 268–69.

Beck, S. L. 1991. The therapeutic use of music for cancer-related pain. *Oncology Nursing Forum* 18 (8): 1327–37.

Cummings, S., and D. Ullman. 1991. *Everybody's Guide to Homeopathic Medicines.* New York: Putnam.

Dossey, B. M., L. Keegan, C. E. Guzzetta, and L. G. Kolkmeier. 1995. *Holistic Nursing: A Handbook for Practice.* 2d ed. Gaithersburg, MD: Aspen.

Frank, J. M. 1985. The effects of music therapy and guided visual imagery on chemotherapy induced nausea and vomiting. *Oncology Nursing Forum* 12 (5): 47–52.

Gould, K. L., D. Ornish, L. Scherwitz, S. Brown, R. P. Edens, M. J. Hess, N. Mullani, F. Dobbs, W. T. Armstrong, T. Merritt, T. Ports, S. Sparier, and J. Billings. 1995. Changes in myocardial perfusion abnormalities by positron emission tomography after long-term, intense risk-factor modification. *Journal of the American Medical Association* 274 (11): 894–901.

Helms, J. 1998. An overview of medical acupuncture. *Alternative Therapies in Health and Medicine* 4 (3): 35–45.

Murray, M. 1996. *Encyclopedia of Nutritional Supplements.* Green Bay, WI: Impakt Communications.

Ornish, D., S. E. Brown, L. W. Scherwitz, J. H. Billings, W. T. Armstrong, T. A. Ports, S. M. McLanahan, R. L. Kirkeeide, R. J. Brand, and K. L. Gould. 1990. Can lifestyle changes reverse coronary heart disease? *The Lancet* 336: 129–33.

Rossman, M. 1987. *Healing Yourself: A Step-by-Step Program for Better Health Through Imagery.* New York: Walker.

Spiegel, D., J. R. Bloom, H. C. Kraemer, et al. 1989. Effect of psychosocial treatment on survival of patients with metastatic breast cancer. *Lancet* 2: 888–91.

Villaire, M. 1998. NIH consensus conference confirms acupuncture's efficacy. *Alternative Therapies in Health and Medicine* 4 (1): 21–22.

Weil, A. 1995. *Natural Health, Natural Medicine.* Boston: Houghton Mifflin.

Wirth, D. P., J. T. Richardson, W. S. Eidelman, and A. C. O'Malley. 1993. Full thickness dermal wounds treated with non-contact therapeutic touch: A replication and extension. *Complementary Therapies in Medicine* 1 (3): 127–32.

Wirth, D. P., M. J. Barrett, and W. S. Eidelman. 1994. Non-contact therapeutic touch and wound re-epithelialization: An extension of previous research. *Complementary Therapies in Medicine* 94 (2): 187–92.

Wirth, D. P., J. T. Richardson, R. D. Martinez, W. S. Eidelman, and M. E. Lopez. 1996. Non-contact therapeutic touch intervention and full-thickness cutaneous wounds: A replication. *Complementary Therapies in Medicine* 2 (4): 237–40.

References

The following excellent resources also were used for the definitions, descriptions, and indications for use for the alternative and complementary therapies included in this chapter:

National Institutes of Health. *Alternative Medicine: Expanding Medical Horizons.* A report to the National Institutes of Health on Alternative Medical Systems and Practices in the United States. Washington, DC: U.S. Government Printing Office, 1992.

Time-Life Books. *The Medical Advisor: The Complete Guide to Alternative and Conventional Treatments.* New York: Time-Life Books, 1996.

Planning an Integrative Health Care Project

The focus of this chapter is on the practical concerns of planning an integrative health care project in an organization or group practice. The planning process is described as a series of 13 steps:

1. Assessing organizational readiness
2. Forming the planning group
3. Developing a budget
4. Establishing goals and objectives
5. Selecting alternative therapies
6. Establishing a credentialing mechanism
7. Planning for resistance
8. Developing a staff training/education plan
9. Developing strategies for risk management
10. Determining structural and environmental needs
11. Maintaining open communication
12. Establishing a timeline
13. Developing a project description

Step 1: Assessing Organizational Readiness

One of the major concerns of any organization is whether it is ready for an integrative health care project. This is important, because if the project begins before the organization is committed to its implementation, the project will probably fail due to opposition. Also, once opposition is strong enough to stop the project, even temporarily, it becomes more difficult to restart it. Following are the key indicators of an organization's readiness to accept an integrative approach:

- Employee attitudes
- Organizational culture
- Community support
- Commitment to project values

Figure 3-1 lists questions that the planning group may use as a guide to determine the organization's readiness to begin an integrative health care project.

Employee Attitudes

Key employees can help the project planning group decide whether the organization is ready to begin an integrative health care project. The administrative team needs to be totally committed to the project. No matter how well planned the project, there will be opposition or resistance, and key administrative staff will need to address concerns and show full support for the project. If those opposing the project sense any reticence from administration, they will know that if they continue the resistance, there is a good chance that the decision to follow an integrative approach can be reversed.

There also needs to be a consensus among the planning group, administration, and the physician/nurse champion(s) concerning which alternative therapies will be integrated into care, at least for the initial project phase. No one can afford to make any comments that the therapies selected are "not the ones they would have chosen" or that they have reservations about certain therapies. All members of the planning group need to be thoroughly educated about alternative and complementary therapies so they can answer questions about and show support for the therapies and the selection rationale.

Key personnel from various departments and clinical services need to agree to participate in the project, even during

FIGURE 3-1. Cues for Assessing Organizational Readiness

- Is the administrative team committed to the project?
- Do all key administrative staff fully support integrative health care?
- Have physician and nurse champions been identified?
- Have members from the major departments agreed to participate on the planning group?
- Has a unit or department agreed to serve as a pilot or demonstration site?
- Is there support in the community for integrative health care? Is there a community member who could serve on the planning group?
- Are the members of the planning group knowledgeable enough about alternative and complementary therapies and their integration to answer questions?
- Does the overall culture of the organization support innovation?
- Does the organization deal well with change, or is it resistant to change?
- Are the resources (people, time, finances) needed for an integrative health care project available?
- Do the current communication processes allow a continuous flow of information to key people in a timely fashion?
- Is there consensus among all concerned parties about which alternative therapies will be integrated?

---

what might be their busy time of the year or short-staffed time of day. This is especially necessary for the departments or services that will be most actively involved in the initial phases of the project. For example, if the oncology unit has agreed to serve as the demonstration unit, full support is needed to ensure that whatever alternative therapies are to be integrated will be incorporated into care even on the weekends or when the unit is a staff member short.

Organizational Culture

The overall culture of the organization needs to be supportive of innovation or a change of this magnitude certainly will not work. One of the ways in which an organization shows that it supports and encourages change is when it continually devotes adequate resources to improvement and development; for example, when monies are included in the organization's budget for optional innovative projects, not just for those projects that are mandated by a governmental or accrediting agency. If, in reviewing the projects undertaken by the organization over the past five years, many innovations have been tried and successfully implemented, it is likely that integrative health care will be successful as well. This is especially true if many of the previous changes either were attempted before many other organizations had already made similar changes or were made in a creative fashion that differed from methods used by other organizations. Organizations in which employees often say, "If it isn't broken, why fix it?" or that only change when the requirements of the Joint Commission on Accreditation of Healthcare Organizations or a state regulatory body require it, are not ideal sites for integrative health care projects at this time.

Another indicator of cultural readiness is an organization's communication processes. If established processes work well—that is, they allow information to flow back and forth between people in a timely fashion—they will enhance the potential for an integrative project to succeed. In organizations with effective communication, staff rarely say that "they had no idea" that change was planned until it happened, or indicate that they could have provided input into planning or implementation but were never asked.

Community Support

Another key indicator for project readiness is that the organization has the support of the community. There may even be a community leader willing to serve as a member of the planning group.

Commitment to Project Values

Models for integrative health care range from one provider incorporating one alternative therapy into his or her practice to entire organizations implementing the integrative health care philosophy as the framework for care in all departments. Although the model used by each organization or group practice depends on its culture, the needs of its community, practitioner qualifications, and budget limitations, certain core values need to underlie any integrative health care program and be held as fundamental by all practitioners and staff. These include a commitment to:

- *Optimal level of health.* Providers believe that integrating alternative and complementary healing therapies with conventional care provides people with a wide array of reputable options for reaching and maintaining an optimal level of health.
- *Partnership between practitioners and patients.* Providing integrated care implies a partnership between practitioners and patients. The notion of partnership is based on the premise that people are responsible for their own health and choices they make that affect their health. They need to be aware of this responsibility and to be provided with complete information about the array of options available to them so they can select those options that will best promote their health. The increased desire for collaboration is driven by both consumers and care practitioners.
- *Use of therapies of least risk as first options.* In integrative care, the least invasive or least risky healing therapies need to be thought of as the first options for care. That is, if a person's condition is not life threatening, a therapy such as acupuncture or homeopathy needs to be tried before more invasive techniques such as surgery or prescription medications. The ideal plan of care is one that integrates options from allopathic care and alternative and complementary care. This type of plan is believed most likely to benefit patients with the least risk and lowest cost possible.
- *A supportive physical environment.* The physical setting in which care is provided needs to support healing and the provider-patient relationship. The context in which integrative health care is provided fosters the health of all who are involved in the project.

Commitment of the planning group and administration to these core values is an important sign of readiness to begin an integrative health care project.

Step 2: Forming the Planning Group

The most important resources needed for an integrative health care project are the people who will provide the leadership for project planning, implementation, and evaluation. Project planning group members include those who will have responsibility for project direction, facilitation or coordination, and communication; staff education/development; and administrative support. The planning group, in concert with administration, determines the project goals and objectives, the organization's readiness for integrative health care, which alternative therapies and providers will be incorporated into care and in what ways, the educational plan for staff and providers, the project timeline and budget, a communication plan, and the resources needed to accomplish these tasks.

Group Size

The initial two or three core members of the planning group are usually selected by administrative leaders; other members can be added when the planning group meets to decide composition. The ideal size for a planning group depends on the size of the organization and the scope of the integrative project. A small group works well for a group practice or a satellite site of a health maintenance organization. A group of seven to eight is usually enough to represent the stakeholders in a large organization. Some complex organizations find that they need as many as 15 to 16 members in their planning group; a group of this size functions more as a steering committee and the work of the group is done in subcommittees.

Representation

The most important consideration other than size when forming the planning group is that of representation. A number of disciplines, departments, units, and leaders need to participate in planning to ensure that the interests and potential contributions of all who work in those areas are taken into account. First, the project planning group needs a physician champion and, if the organization is a large one with nursing staff, a nurse champion as well. In addition to the physician and nurse champions, the planning group will need the involvement of such disciplines or departments in the organization as social services, pharmacy, staff development or education, employee health, and physical therapy. Physicians and nurses from various clinical services need to be included as well.

Since most successful projects in organizations are multidisciplinary in nature, as are activities related to patient care, it is best to have representation from as many key disciplines and departments as possible. Moreover, an effort needs to be made to keep the focus on the multidisciplinary or consumer focus of the project, so the project is not used for a single department to meet its own needs. At the initial planning group meetings, each person's role in project development, implementation, and evaluation needs to be discussed. Most members of the group will be involved in all phases of the project, but some may be more involved in one phase than another. For example, a researcher or statistician will have more involvement in the evaluation phase than in the other aspects of the project.

Selection of the Project Director or Coordinator

Of primary concern is the selection or appointment of the person who will have overall responsibility for the project, directing or coordinating the effort and addressing the questions or concerns that will arise throughout. The ideal director would have both vision and good managerial skills—a difficult combination to find. This role requires expertise in organization and communication combined with a broad understanding of the organization's vision and resources. If a choice needs to be made between a visionary and a managerial expert, the best choice for the project director position would most likely be the person with vision. It is essential, though, in this case, that an assistant with project management experience or first-line managerial experience be appointed. The major role of the project director or coordinator is to ensure that the important tasks in the planning process are accomplished.

The project director is responsible for keeping top-level administrators apprised of progress, ensuring that actions are consistent with the goals of the organization and in accord with the specific, written goals and objectives developed for the integrative health care program. Although the director may need a good deal of latitude in performing the role, an effective oversight mechanism on the legality of all activities needs to exist. Although such a mechanism does not guarantee freedom from litigation and/or censure from the conventional medical community, without such safeguards it is difficult to withstand the inevitable assaults from the conventional establishment or to ensure a confident patient population.

Meeting Frequency

The planning group needs to decide the frequency of its meetings, depending on the scope of the project and the need for group discussion; the frequency can vary throughout the course of the project. It is typical for planning groups to meet weekly in the beginning of the planning phase because so many decisions need to be made; as the project progresses into the implementation phase, monthly or even quarterly meetings may be sufficient. The need for frequent face-to-face meetings depends on the degree of comfort that group members have with each other and whether the organization has the capability to provide for long-distance meetings and communication via teleconferences, videoconferences, or e-mail. Although the planning group needs to have frequent in-person meetings, it is important for the project director to monitor the content of each meeting and how much progress is being made. When groups meet just for the sake of meeting, no matter how exciting the vision may be, the meetings are perceived as a waste of time and attendance begins to decrease. It is important to remember that meetings should keep people informed, facilitate decision making, and allow all of those involved in the project to provide input. With this in mind, meetings and communication can take place via the most convenient method or media.

Acquisition of Relevant Information

There are several ways the planning group can acquire information on which to base its plans. The most common are literature review, conference attendance and networking, use of consultants, visits to other organizations that have already implemented an integrative health care program, and educational courses.

Literature Review

A critical review of the literature to get up-to-date information concerning any reports of integrative health care projects and any outcome data can be helpful to the planning group as it begins its work. Both alternative therapy and mainstream journals have reports of integrative health care projects and publish research regarding alternative therapies. Many sites that conduct and publish research in this area also have clinical practice areas. Especially helpful are the names of authors who are familiar with these types of projects and may have experience in settings similar to the planning group's organization. Most are willing to share their experiences with others. Obtaining information from those who have already implemented and evaluated such a project can be crucial in the planning phase.

Conference Attendance and Networking

Key members of the planning group and administrative staff can attend conferences and meetings that will help to stimulate their thinking about which alternative and complementary therapies to begin integrating. At those gatherings they will meet many people with whom they can network, finding out what others have done in various sites. They will find people generally very open to sharing plans they implemented that did or did not work. Many even will have developed strategies that your organization or group practice could use based on their experience.

Overall, discussing the experiences of others can help the group members to achieve consensus on the important areas to address in this type of project. Contact with other organizations and their planning groups can provide a support network, as well as valuable information, evaluation forms, and outcome measures. Modifying the policies, procedures, forms, and evaluation tools of others is much easier and more cost-effective than developing them from scratch.

Professional Consultants

Attending conferences can also provide the names of those who may be of value to the organization in a consulting capacity. Expert consultants who have experience in integrative health care projects can help in deciding which project elements need the most emphasis, showing how other organizations decided which alternative therapies to incorporate, and providing external support for selected therapies. Consultants can help to answer specific questions concerning how an integrative model might be adapted to an organization's goals and objectives.

Site Visits

It is difficult to know whether it is worthwhile to spend the time and money necessary to visit an organization(s). Certainly, there is some inspirational value in having the planning group see firsthand what other programs have done and what other sites "feel" like. However, some members will be disappointed if they find that the place they are visiting does not look any different than their own facility. In many instances, the differences lie not as much in how a place looks or feels, but in how providers view and practice health care.

Educational Opportunities

In general, courses sponsored by credible journals, universities and other not-for-profit groups are usually very helpful. Many schools of medicine and nursing, and public health, health management, dentistry, and other health care professional schools offer both formal and continuing education courses in integrating alternative and complementary therapies into practice. Many continuing education courses have gained the approval of an accrediting body, such as the American Medical Association, the American Nurses' Association, or a similar professional group.

Step 3: Developing a Budget

The next task of the planning group is to develop a budget. During the planning phase, budget parameters are needed to determine appropriate goals and objectives. All current and projected activities—whether or not they are already being performed by someone in the organization—need to be included, and time and materials costs need to be considered in addition to straight monetary costs. For example, even if those who will educate staff are already on salary, the costs of their time and any new educational materials need to be allocated to the project. Costs for other resources may include library research; consultants; preparation of the final project report, posters, and presentations in various media; and preparation of articles describing the organization's experiences in project development, implementation, and evaluation. It is important to break out individual program components because it is difficult to determine the actual costs of planning, implementing, and evaluating a project when many expenses remain hidden. Actual costs, not estimates, should be used whenever possible. An overview of budget elements for the planning, implementation, and evaluation phases of an integrative health care project is provided in chapter 6.

Some organizations have reduced certain costs by having student personnel incorporate parts of the integrative health care project efforts into school requirements. For example, students in master's and doctoral programs can analyze outcome data generated by organization projects as the basis for a thesis or dissertation.

Step 4: Establishing Goals and Objectives

Establishing the goals and objectives the organization wants to achieve is the next step in the planning phase. It is essential that these be developed by a multidisciplinary group from as many of the affected settings and departments as possible, because this will help achieve "buy in." The goals and objectives need to be seen as essential by senior management, administration, and the board of directors because these are the people who will need to answer questions about the reasons for the organization's involvement in such a project and provide the resources needed for project success. Goals and objectives are important for strategic planning because they state both the overall purpose for the project and the specific outcomes it intends to achieve.

Project Goals

Goals are the broad aims of the integrative health care project. Some examples might be:

- To improve the quality of health care in the community
- To increase the health care options available to patients and the community
- To better meet the diverse needs of the cultures served

Goals are not intended to be measured, but rather to provide a framework to help those in the organization remember the larger purpose for which the project is being developed.

Project Objectives

Objectives are specific outcomes the organization expects to achieve after integrative health care is implemented. They are concrete statements that are both realistic and measurable. The objectives are what will be used to determine whether integrative health care has been implemented successfully in the organization. By answering the following questions, the planning group may collect useful information for developing organization-specific objectives:

- What outcomes are desired from this project?
- What will be different within the organization after integrative health care is implemented?
- What will be different about what patients, staff, and/or the community know, do, or feel after integrative health care is implemented?
- What changes in cost, quality of care, or satisfaction are expected after project implementation?
- How long will it take for these changes to occur?
- Are the expected changes realistic given the budgetary constraints?

This information is important because, although many organizations are developing integrative health care projects, the reasons for that development may be very different. For example, one organization may institute such a project to improve patient satisfaction with its services, whereas another may adopt integrative health care to improve its market share or to meet the demands of its main third-party payer. It is important to remember that project objectives measure the degree to which *outcomes* of the project were achieved (described in chapter 5), not the degree to which the *project itself* was implemented (described in chapter 4).

When developing project objectives, planning group members and administrative staff need to determine the outcome measures that will be used to evaluate whether the project has achieved its desired objectives. For example, if one of the project objectives is to increase patient satisfaction with pain management, an outcome measure that will be used to evaluate the degree to which the objective is met also needs to be selected. Figure 3-2 shows a sample statement of objectives.

All objectives and outcome measures need to be realistic based on the organization's available resources, culture, and time frame for implementation and evaluation (discussed in step 12). For example, identifying an outcome measure that will

---

FIGURE 3-2. Sample Statement of Objectives for an Integrative Health Care Project

Six months after implementation of the integrative health care project, the following objectives will have been accomplished:

- There will be an increase of at least 10 percent in overall patient satisfaction with care, as measured by random telephone audits of discharged patients.
- At least 15 percent of the community will view this facility as being progressive, as measured by the quarterly marketing survey.
- At least 20 percent of the community will be aware that alternative and complementary therapies are integrated into conventional care at this facility, as measured by the quarterly marketing survey.
- There will be a decrease of at least 10 percent in costs for laboratory services at this facility for all categories of patient care.
- There will be an increase of at least 20 percent in patient satisfaction with pain management, as measured on the patient discharge satisfaction with care survey.

---

require nurses to interview patients may be too labor-intensive for an organization with a limited number of staff. Likewise, if a project objective is to increase community awareness of the organization's move to integrative health care by 25 percent, it is unlikely that this objective can be achieved in a six-month period. More detailed information regarding evaluation of project objectives and selection of appropriate outcome measures is provided in chapter 5.

Step 5: Selecting Alternative Therapies

The planning group's next task is to select which alternative and complementary therapies will be integrated with conventional care and in what order. For example, group members need to discuss whether they wish to begin integration with therapies such as imagery and Therapeutic Touch that are unlikely to have side effects, or whether the fact that a well-respected physician on staff is also an expert in acupuncture might positively influence other practitioners' acceptance of the project as a whole. The physician and nurse champions can be very helpful in these decisions because of their knowledge of alternative therapies and the needs of the organization's patient population.

To select the therapies on an objective basis, and not just on staff members' preferences, guidelines need to be developed. Criteria to be applied to each therapy under consideration include:

- Degree of risk
- Usefulness to the patient population served
- Availability of expertise
- Length of time needed to prepare competent practitioners
- Any scope of practice restrictions
- Additional patient care time needed to implement the therapy

Group members then need to determine how the selected therapies will be integrated. The two major options are to integrate therapies within an existing program or to develop a new program devoted solely to integrative care. For example, meditation, herbal remedies, and acupuncture can be incorporated within an existing pain management program or set up under a separate department of alternative and complementary therapies. The most common option is to begin by incorporating therapies into existing programs. This method of integration achieves several purposes:

- It sends an immediate message that the organization is committed to keeping the best of conventional care, but wishes to provide more options for patients and providers.
- It allows time for providers to become competent in selected therapies.
- It allows the organization to begin the integration project slowly, which increases the likelihood of its success. This is because allowing more time can permit everyone who wishes to be involved to become familiar with selected therapies— and with the idea of integrative care.

Limiting initial integration to one, two, or three alternative therapies permits the gradual introduction of alternative therapies and is a more logical decision if practitioners need to be educated in the new therapies. If an organization is too ambitious and tries to institute an integrative health care program with many therapies all at one time, practitioners have insufficient time to become competent in either all of the alternative therapies or in ways of integrating these therapies into conventional care. Even practitioners who are not actually providing the therapies need preparation time so they can answer questions posed by patients or the community.

Examples of existing programs in which alternative therapies can be integrated include the following: patient/community education, quality improvement programs, pain management programs, chronic illness support groups, well-child care centers, health promotion programs, stress management programs, research and experimental projects, hospice/palliative care, continuing education programs, and healing environment or Planetree projects.

The programs listed work well for beginning integrative efforts because they are accepted conventional projects that already exist, thereby eliminating the politics that occur in any organization when a new project is proposed. Also, many of these care programs can benefit from increasing the array of options presented to patients. For example, those who facilitate chronic illness support groups (such as for diabetes or cardiovascular problems) often wish that they had more treatment suggestions for managing symptoms. Continuing education and research projects that use alternative therapies and their integration as a focus are considered more interesting by many staff; the therapies benefit not only the patients and their families, but also the staff.

As with other patient care protocols, policies and procedures for alternative therapies and their use need to be written; these policies and procedures need to follow the same format and guidelines as do others. State rules and regulations for the practice of each therapy need to be examined. For example, verification of which therapies are within the scope of practice of each discipline is important; in some states, acupuncture may be considered within the scope of medical, but not nursing, practice. Also, many states require acupuncturists to be licensed, and three states require physicians who practice homeopathy to be licensed by a state board of homeopathic medical examiners.

Step 6: Establishing a Credentialing Mechanism

One major challenge in the planning phase is finding physicians and nurses who are expert in one or more alternative therapies and who view their practice as integrative. There are some providers whose practice is mainly conventional health care, but who provide one or two alternative therapies. These providers do not necessarily view their practice as integrative; they see themselves as providing primarily conventional care. Still other physicians or nurses are competent in the practice of alternative or complementary therapies and view their practice as solely alternative; they do not practice conventional care. The ideal providers for an integrative health care project are those who are competent in an array of both conventional and alternative therapies, do not see the two types of care as mutually exclusive, and can offer patients the most appropriate choices in either category.

Just as the qualifications of practitioners are critiqued for conventional care, the planning group needs to identify the needed education/training and experience for providers of alternative therapies. This is necessary even for those practitioners such as nurses or physicians whose qualifications for conventional care have been reviewed. One of the major reasons for the credentialing process is to permit the group practice or organization to advertise that the providers of alternative and complementary therapies associated with them are truly qualified to practice those therapies. Also, it is easier to seek reimbursement for the services of alternative therapy practitioners who are credentialed in some fashion, because insurers are more comfortable that such providers are credible.

The credentialing process begins by identifying the basic conventional educational or training preparation needed to practice a specific alternative therapy. For example, an organization may choose to restrict the practice of acupuncture to allopathic, osteopathic, or naturopathic physicians and nurse practitioners, rather than permitting any acupuncturist to go through the credentialing process. In contrast, a group practice may determine that a provider of guided imagery does not need educational background in any of the health professions.

Next, the planning group needs to check with the state boards and professional organizations for information concerning the scope of practice of health professionals in their state and any advisory opinions related to the practice of alternative therapies. For example, some states have issued advisory opinions that Therapeutic Touch is within the scope of practice for registered nurses. State licensing requirements for the alternative therapies or healing systems also should be identified. For example, many states require acupuncturists to be licensed, while others do not have any regulations governing acupuncture. Also, some states license naturopathic medical practice, while others do not. The educational requirements for practitioners of selected alternative therapies are covered in chapter 2 and relevant organizations are listed in appendix A.

The planning group next determines minimum education and experience requirements. For example, the group may require that physicians practicing acupuncture need to have completed the medical acupuncture program sponsored by the University of California–Los Angeles or an equivalent program and 100 hours of practice prior to approval to practice acupuncture. Similarly, the planning group could require that anyone who wants to integrate Therapeutic Touch into conventional care needs to have attended, at a minimum, a one-day workshop facilitated by a teacher approved as a member of the Teachers Cooperative of Nurse Healers–Professional Associates International, Inc. or have his or her practice reviewed and approved by a member of that association. The planning group also needs to determine reasonable requirements for continuing education and annual experience for practitioners to maintain their credentials to practice specific therapies.

Overall, the credentialing process for alternative therapies is no different in principle than the process for conventional health care. It can seem more challenging at times, because the educational and training requirements for many alternative therapies are not as standardized as are those for conventional care.

Step 7: Planning for Resistance

It is important that integrative health care be seen as a unified program and not as business as usual with a few alternative therapies added. Integration of these therapies into conventional care requires a different mind set on the part of most practitioners and administrators who have been educated in the current allopathic or conventional care paradigm—that perspective is not all-inclusive enough to allow alternative therapies to be an easy fit.

Many people involved in and with the organization may respond negatively to the idea of integrating alternative therapies into conventional care. It is crucial in the planning phase to identify those people who may be resistant to the project and on what reasoning or viewpoint they are likely to base their position. This way, potential strategies to deal with their expressed and unexpressed concerns can be developed prior to project implementation. (Additional strategies to deal with resistance to implementing an integrative health care project can be found in chapter 4.)

The planning group needs to plan for ways to help change the existing mind set of those who resist change to an integrative system, which eventually may require a commitment to the integration of all valid therapies into all patient care efforts. It is important to include leaders from administration and various departments and services in this planning, because their commitment to the project will be essential in dealing with future resistance.

Step 8: Developing a Staff Training/ Education Plan

One of the most important integrative health care project activities is that of educating those inside and outside the organization about alternative and complementary therapies. In the United States, there are few direct care staff, and almost no support personnel, who are knowledgeable and skilled in any of the alternative therapies. In addition, those staff who are competent in the use of an alternative therapy may not be skilled in integrating that therapy with conventional care or in teaching others about the modality or its integration. If staff feel that, because the organization is integrating alternative therapies, it is permissible for them to practice any alternative therapy they wish, the overall progress of the project can be hampered. All efforts need to be seen as part of an integrative project and not as the practice of separate alternative therapies.

An examination of existing training programs can help the planning group to determine which educational efforts are appropriate to provide staff with the preparation they need for practice of specific alternative therapies and ways to integrate those therapies into practice. Some programs can be provided in the organizational setting and others will require staff travel to conferences or seminars. Training programs are also offered on-line or through other long-distance learning methods. It is usually helpful to plan to educate a small group in each alternative therapy selected, rather than training one or two staff members in many therapies. Small-group training fosters the development of a supportive network among practitioners and keeps an organization's efforts from becoming scattered.

Organizations and conferences that provide training programs in alternative therapies and integrating them into conventional care can be found in appendix A.

Step 9: Developing Strategies for Risk Management

As the number of alternative therapies and providers increases, so do the liability concerns and, in turn, the need to use a variety of mechanisms to decrease the risk involved. The most commonly used are credentialing, organizationwide education and training, and effective documentation.

Credentialing

One of the most important risk management strategies is that of provider credentialing, which was discussed in step 6. Most essential in this process from a risk management perspective is the need to review and document the preparation of providers and to determine the therapies that are within the scope of practice. New legislation is being passed on an almost daily basis, and it is important to stay abreast of any changes in law.

Education and Training

Second in importance is the provision of extensive education and training for everyone in the organization or group practice concerning applicable alternative therapies and concerns that may arise when those therapies are used in combination with conventional therapies. Even though a practitioner may be an excellent massage therapist, for example, he or she needs to know that massage therapy is not recommended within 24 hours after acupuncture because it can reverse the healing process. Similarly, providers may be very knowledgeable concerning herbal preparations and nutritional supplements, but they need to know that recommending garlic can increase bleeding time (as can some conventional medications) and should not be used in conjunction with many medications. All providers, whether or not they integrate alternative therapies, need to ask patients which alternative therapies they are using and be able to answer general questions they may be asked about those therapies. Assessment and intake forms need to include use of alternative therapies as well.

Documentation

As in conventional care, documentation of all aspects of alternative therapy education and treatment is essential. Detailed, accurate records of education, training, licensure, and any certifications need to be kept. It is wise, as well, to work closely with malpractice liability providers as alternative therapies are integrated. A detailed review of the legal aspects of integrative health care is provided in chapter 7.

Step 10: Determining Structural and Environmental Needs

One of the most common misconceptions among those considering an integrative health care project is that major changes to the current physical structure will be needed. Usually, few changes are necessary; the plan for any changes can be made on the basis of the financial resources available for the project. Most organizations that have implemented integrative health care projects report that, even if they made major alterations in the physical facilities, they are unsure they would devote the resources to those changes if they had it to do over.

The changes that seem important are those that give people a sense that they are in an organization with a culture that supports healing. Walls that are painted in soft colors and rooms that have soft lighting facilitate a healing environment without much expense. Appropriate artwork can be provided in many instances by community artists or organization staff who are artists in their nonwork time. Music can be made available using inexpensive radios or CD players; music serves the dual purpose of relaxing people and serving as a buffer for extraneous noise that is present in any busy organization. Plants or rock gardens are preferred over flowers or floral arrangements because many people are sensitive to scents. Simple modifications, such as using wood armoires instead of steel cabinets for supplies, can add much to the "human" feel of a facility.

Planning for a group practice that is not physically incorporated into a large organization can be kept simple as well. There is no need to have a large number of providers at one fancy location. It is advisable for each location to have two to three physicians and nurse providers. Ancillary personnel, such as those who provide guided imagery or massage therapy, can have hours there as needed or can provide care at separate locations. Several smaller sites that are geographically convenient for consumers are usually more beneficial than one large facility. Having several smaller sites allows a large umbrella organization to remain flexible.

Step 11: Maintaining Open Communication

Communication is one of the most important activities during all phases of the project, but especially during the planning phase. This is because no matter how much information concerning the project the planning group disseminates, there will be people who will say they were never informed regarding what was planned. Because a project that integrates alternative therapies can be considered different from more mainstream ones, it is better that the project be perceived by staff and the community as an open one—that is, that there is no attempt to hide any information. Unless accurate information is disseminated on a frequent and consistent basis, rumors are likely to flourish. Also, many who wish to be involved in the project may not be able to be of assistance in the early phases if they do not know about the project. Many health care providers do not make it common knowledge that they are competent in one or more alternative therapies.

Keeping records of the activities of the planning group and communicating those records to the rest of the organization are essential functions. It is best if one person has responsibility for record keeping and communication; that person needs to have excellent writing skills, record all pertinent activities concisely, and distribute meeting minutes in a timely manner. If possible, it is best to have someone who is not involved with the content or direction of the meeting be responsible for recording activities. Staff members who will provide secretarial and clerical support for communication activities also need to be identified.

A mechanism to answer questions about the project should be arranged; a box or voice-mail line can be made available for this purpose. In addition, it is helpful to develop a method for keeping files on activities that seemingly have little or nothing to do with the project, but can have an effect on project implementation and outcomes in the evaluation phase. Examples of activities or events that need to be tracked are reorganization of a department or a patient care unit, changes in management or staff, organization activities, and major changes in the demographics of the community.

Step 12: Establishing a Timeline

When considering the implementation of an integrative health care project, the planning group needs a plan that extends over at least three years. Change of this magnitude takes time. All the people involved, both inside and outside of the organization, need to participate in the planning phase. Although it takes longer to involve everyone, it ensures a more successful project.

Planning time is difficult to estimate, because the amount needed varies according to the needs of the organization and the readiness of the people involved to begin the project. It is frequently very exciting to be involved in this type of project, but not as exciting to attend meetings to work out the details. This can be difficult for the planning group to understand, because members are usually the people in the organization who find change exciting and are the "early adopters" of any innovation. It is important to make a list of all project implementation and evaluation activities. Based on this information, a flowchart can be developed to track the progress of the project throughout all phases.

Time needed for implementation and evaluation is frequently underestimated. Although there is no certain way to predict what factors will slow implementation, there will be delays. For example, some of the staff who have been fully trained in alternative therapies and their integration may leave and their replacements will need training time, and once replacement staff are trained, it may seem as if the project is beginning anew because the previous progress has been lost. Time for the evaluation of outcomes and ongoing monitoring also needs to be included in the plan. Data need to be collected, recorded, and analyzed, and related activities cannot be rushed without compromising the accuracy and dependability of the results. More detailed information regarding data collection and evaluation issues is provided in chapter 5.

Most important, the time needed for planning, implementation, and evaluation phases needs to be in proportion to the scope of the project and the desired outcomes. If an organization introduces one or two alternative therapies into an existing program, less time will be needed in each phase than for a project that integrates six alternative therapies throughout all services in the same organization. Likewise, if the organization desires modest outcomes from integrating alternative therapies, less time needs to be allocated for planning and implementation activities. For example, if the organization wishes to increase patient satisfaction with pain management by 10 percent by the end of six months, less time is needed than if the objective were an increase of 35 percent.

Step 13: Developing a Project Description

One of the main responsibilities of the planning group is the development of a concise description of the integrative health care project. This may be termed a "hallway" or "meeting" description; that is, a description that can be given to someone while walking down the hall or as an overview during a meeting. The description needs to include elements that are important to those in the organization who will be affected by the project. Important questions to consider when developing this description include:

- What type of integrative health care project is planned?
- Exactly how will the methods for providing care change? Exactly what will stay the same?

- Which alternative or complementary therapies will be integrated? Why were those therapies selected?
- Who will provide each therapy, and why were those providers chosen? Will everyone eventually be expected to provide them?
- Who will be in charge of the project? Why was this person selected?
- Who will participate in project planning? Are any specific departments or services excluded and, if so, why?
- Why does this project need to occur? Why is it so important?
- Why does this project need to be planned, implemented, and/or evaluated now? Why can't the organization wait?
- How will this project be implemented? Who will be involved in its implementation? Which departments, shifts, and personnel will be affected and in what sequence?
- When will the project start? Is that date negotiable? When will the project end? Will it end on a specific date? Does a specific change need to occur before the project ends?
- Is this a pilot project or a demonstration project?
- What is the setting for this project? Where will it be implemented? Is only one unit or one group practice going to implement it? How is project implementation going to be monitored?
- How will the project be evaluated? What methods will be used to measure outcomes? What will happen if the project does what is expected? What will happen if it does not do what is expected? What may happen if this project is not implemented?
- How will staff who are not actively involved be kept informed concerning what is going on in the project and its outcomes?

A sample project description is provided in figure 3-3.

Writing a project description serves several purposes. It provides a clear description of all components for anyone who wishes that information, and it ensures that everyone receives firsthand, accurate information. Many times, staff or community members receive distorted information about a project, mainly because they are hearing someone else's interpretation of what was heard at a meeting. It is also of major benefit to the planning group and administration. Often those who serve as part of a planning group believe that all members are "on the same wavelength" or are under the impression that certain

FIGURE 3-3. Sample Project Description

The XYZ Health Care System is planning an integrative health care project that will have the improvement of inpatient pain management as its initial focus. The project will begin by integrating the alternative and complementary therapies of imagery, acupressure, and therapeutic touch into the care currently provided to oncology patients. These therapies were selected because of their low risk to patients, the brief amount of time needed to provide them to patients, and the short time period needed for staff to learn how to provide them and begin incorporating them into care. A core group of nurses on the two oncology units will be trained in the initial phase; all nurses will be expected to incorporate these therapies within a six-month period.

Our goal is that in three years we will be integrating appropriate alternative and complementary therapies throughout the organization. To begin this process, at the same time as the oncology project begins, we will begin an educational program for all staff so they can become knowledgeable about the alternative and complementary therapies our patients are using.

Mary Miller will serve as project director; Mary has extensive experience in facilitating large projects in our system and practices several alternative and complementary therapies. Although personnel from all departments are welcome to participate in the planning phase, representatives from the physician staff, social services, staff development, and marketing will join nursing in the beginning efforts. If any department, employee, or provider wishes to be involved in the planning efforts, please contact Mary.

We are beginning this project for many reasons, the most important of which is that our patients can benefit from the use of these therapies. Community leaders are asking us to continue to provide excellent conventional care while incorporating some of the valid alternative therapies. We need to maintain our commitment to our patients that we will provide progressive, high-quality health care, and integrative health care is one way for us to do that.

The project will begin with a core group of nurses on oncology representing all shifts. The planning group, in consultation with administration, will decide the sequence of implementing integrative health care on other units and departments. The project will begin on October 1. We will monitor implementation on an ongoing basis using a tool that has been developed for that purpose.

We will measure patients' pain management and their satisfaction with our integrative efforts. We will use a visual analogue scale to determine how well we are managing patient pain and a measure of patient satisfaction with the program that was specifically designed for this project. We will monitor the results of both measures on a monthly basis and communicate those results first to the staff on the oncology unit and then in our system's newsletter.

decisions have been made. Putting the main project elements in writing allows a review of that information by all group members; misperceptions can be clarified before distribution.

Conclusion

The series of steps provided in this chapter follows the process of planning an integrative health care project in an organization or group practice. It can be used as a guide by administrative staff, the project director, and planning group members throughout this phase of development. The next chapter focuses on ways of monitoring project implementation and strategies to deal with issues that arise during the implementation phase.

Implementing an Integrative Health Care Project

T his chapter focuses on the three most important factors to be considered during the implementation phase of project development: monitoring, minimization of conflict, and communication. The importance of each of these factors is discussed, as are the essential components of an implementation monitoring plan, strategies for dealing with opposition, and ways to ensure effective communication. These factors are key to project success, and, as stated in chapter 3, sufficient time must be allotted for each of them.

The Importance of Implementation Monitoring

Most often when a project fails to achieve the expected results, it is because the project elements were not implemented as designed. However, most organizations do not monitor the actual implementation of a project. Commonly, data concerning project outcomes may be collected for evaluation (see chapter 5), but no concrete information is available to help determine the status of implementation. Most organizations rely solely on the perceptions of administrators or managers to determine whether a project is being implemented as originally planned.

Revising the Timeline

Because an integrative health care project can take several years for implementation, it helps the planning group to know which stage of implementation has been reached at any one time. Based on status information, group members will be able to tell whether the project is proceeding according to the time frame developed during the planning phase. A distinct deviation from the timeline may indicate that original estimates were overly ambitious and should be revised for the rest of the project. It also may signal the need for changing the methods of implementation originally established or providing help in areas where progress is lacking.

Adapting the Original Plan

Status information is important not only because the organization needs to know how far the project has progressed at key intervals, but also because the information can be used to make any needed changes in the plan. Knowing that one unit or department is not where it needs to be in implementing integrative health care helps the planning group and managers to make any changes that might be needed to facilitate progress in that area. Often, help is not provided where required until the outcome data are analyzed in the evaluation phase and it is noticed that some areas had worse outcomes than others.

It is helpful to know which alternative and complementary therapies are being implemented with little difficulty; the planning group can use this information as the project expands to other units, departments, or practices. If some healing therapies are meeting opposition or staff members are having more difficulty using them with a specific patient population, that is useful information as well. If a cardiac care unit is having difficulty integrating imagery, for example, it is beneficial to help the staff determine why that is so. Perhaps imagery is not a therapy that the staff on that unit are able to teach, or it could be that to be effective imagery needs to be taught before surgery rather than after. Analyzing implementation information allows the planning group to make a knowledgeable decision concerning whether it is appropriate to continue to try to implement imagery or not—and whether different strategies to implement the therapy are needed for that unit.

Supporting Evaluation Data

Often, an organization reports that its staff has tried to integrate alternative therapies but it "just didn't work," so the project was abandoned. This usually means that evaluation of the project showed poor outcomes without showing why this was so. Perhaps the project was implemented as planned and the outcomes were poor because the plan itself needed revision. Alternatively, implementation may not have followed the plan at all, and the organization would have achieved expected outcomes if it had been. Often key elements stipulated by the planning group or administration are never put into practice, in which case, outcomes are likely to be poor. The organization needs the information provided by implementation monitoring to support and explain the results of evaluation.

Communicating Progress

Monitoring information also can be beneficial in planning celebrations of progress. Progress can be rewarded when a unit or area has achieved a milestone, as demonstrated during the monitoring process, rather than waiting until the entire project is completed. In addition, using scaling methods to monitor implementation (specific methods are described in steps 5 and 6 below) provides objective measures of progress. This information is helpful when the planning group wants to communicate what is happening in specific departments, units, or areas to the rest of the organization.

Development of a Monitoring Plan

Because implementation monitoring is so important to the success of an integrative health care project, the monitoring plan must be carefully and fully developed. The details of identifying

what should be monitored, by what method(s), and by whom
are provided in the following eight steps:

1. Identifying the essential project components
2. Monitoring the involvement of key people
3. Tracking project time frames
4. Recording organizational events
5. Monitoring the degree of implementation
6. Monitoring staff perceptions
7. Developing procedures for collecting and reviewing information
8. Determining monitoring frequency

Step 1: Identifying the Essential Project Components

The first and most important step in developing the monitoring
plan is to create a checklist of the project components to be
monitored, including therapies and philosophy, and the degree
of change expected for each. This checklist should be made at
the beginning of the implementation phase.

Identifying the essential components to be monitored during implementation is important because unless those elements
are actually implemented, the project may not be successful.
For example, an integrative health care project may be planned
for implementation on an oncology unit and is to integrate
acupuncture, Therapeutic Touch, and guided imagery. If only
two of the three alternative therapies are actually integrated,
the same outcomes may not be achieved as would be possible
if all three had been implemented. The checklist of elements,
then, helps to make sure that all of the essential components
that contribute to project success are included in the monitoring process.

Therapies

The most essential project components to be included on the
checklist are the alternative therapies that the planning group
and administration decided to integrate on each unit. For example, imagery and Therapeutic Touch may be planned for

integration on one unit, while imagery and acupressure may be planned for another unit with a different patient population.

Philosophy and Practice

If a change in philosophy is expected in addition to the integration of specific alternative therapies, then that change needs to be added to the checklist of project elements. For example, if staff are supposed to begin viewing their practice as a partnership with patients, then that element needs to be on the checklist. This is because, in addition to monitoring whether imagery is being integrated into care for the postoperative patient group, monitoring of implementation needs to include whether or not staff members' attitudes toward practice have changed. Monitoring attitudes may mean analyzing documentation of care provided: staff who view care as a partnership will document that they have discussed a variety of care options with patients, while those with a conventional viewpoint will document what they "did" for a patient. If monitoring that change in philosophy is not on the initial checklist of elements, it is less likely to be done.

Degree of Implementation

The checklist of essential project elements should include the degree to which those elements are expected to be implemented. For example, if Therapeutic Touch was to be learned and used by all of the registered nurses on the oncology unit, and only four nurses did so, then even though Therapeutic Touch was implemented, it was not used to the extent expected. If the integrative health care project is not implemented as planned, or not implemented to the extent planned, outcomes will be affected.

Step 2: Monitoring the Involvement of Key People

A checklist of the people, departments, services, or disciplines expected to participate in each phase of the project needs to be made. Certain disciplines or individuals are critical in all phases of the project, while others are needed only in one phase.

Physicians and nurses, for example, need to participate in all phases, yet representatives from marketing or medical records may only be involved in the planning or evaluation phases. Those who were essential in the planning phase, such as administrators, may be less directly involved in some of the implementation activities. Also, in some organizations, departments such as human resources are included in all phases of any project. If that is the case, even though the planning group only needs the involvement of the human resources department for a specific purpose, such as position description revisions, that department needs to be included in all phases to increase the likelihood of project success.

It is important to identify clearly those who need to be integrally involved in implementation from the very beginning of this phase, so that continual monitoring of their involvement can be done. Frequently, those who complain later that they did not have a say in what was happening or did not get to give their input when change was occurring are those who did not participate actively during the planning or implementation phases. Active participation by key people is important in any project, but becomes more so with an integrative health care project. This is because the therapies provided are outside of mainstream care, so providers and staff are unfamiliar with them. Also, changes in awareness of what the project is all about occur subtly, and those who miss planning group or subcommittee meetings will be left behind.

Step 3: Tracking Project Time Frames

Another key element of the implementation monitoring plan is the identification of whether the project and its elements begin on time and are proceeding as planned. The specific accomplishments that need to be completed on a monthly or quarterly basis are used to develop a monitoring checklist. The essential project elements identified in step 1 and the key people who need to be involved as identified in step 2 are used as the basis for this checklist. Time frames for each of those elements and people are identified. For example, if the two previous steps identify that at least three nurses on each unit need to integrate imagery into the care of their patients, a time frame in which that is expected to occur is determined.

Time Frame Variations

Those who participate in the project need to know how much variation in the time frame is permitted. If implementation of a specific component such as acupressure or imagery is expected to occur within six months of project implementation, then staff and managers need to know if that time frame is negotiable. If it is, they need to know what reasons are considered legitimate for adjusting the expected target dates. Those who are key in the implementation phase then need to be held accountable for meeting project time frames. This is important because many staff, providers, and managers have learned through experience that if deadlines or target dates are missed, there are often no repercussions. Indeed, in many instances, if implementation of an unwanted change can be delayed long enough, sometimes the proposed change need never take place.

Variations in Implementation Progress

One of the most noticeable issues that arises during implementation is that, although the overall plan may be designed on the assumption that all areas will progress simultaneously, it is actually rare that they will do so. One area may seem more supportive of integrating alternative therapies than others, and that unit may get off to a rapid start. It is not unusual, however, for such an area to run into implementation difficulties that were not planned and, without appropriate support, staff may get discouraged. Another area may get off to a very slow start and seem to be taking too long to begin making progress, then experience smooth and steady improvement once implementation is under way. A certain amount of speed is important for staff to see the project as a unified one, but a unit that moves too rapidly in the beginning may leave itself open to backlash from those who do not want it to move that quickly.

Step 4: Recording Organizational Events

It is important to develop a system for recording and monitoring events that occur during project implementation that could have an impact on the project itself or the time frame for implementation. For example, changes at any level of system or facility administrative or managerial structure can have a major impact on implementation. Reorganization at one facility and not another may help to explain why implementation went more smoothly at a specific facility in a system. Occurrences such as the departure of a much respected unit manager, a seasonal opening or closing of a unit or department, or the illness of one partner in a group practice are not directly related to essential project elements, but can affect implementation. Even major weather events or local school board conflicts can leave staff with less energy to devote to project implementation. These events and incidents can lead to lack of progress or deviations from planned progress.

Keeping track of these events gives the planning group and administration a basis for assessing implementation monitoring information. For example, when reviewing slower than expected implementation progress on an oncology unit, a record of events might show that the unit manager left two weeks after implementation began, necessitating delays.

Step 5: Monitoring the Degree of Implementation

It is important to know not only whether or not the project is being implemented, but also to what stage the implementation has progressed. Using a scale to record progress is the most efficient means of monitoring degree of implementation. Otherwise, areas will progress at varying rates or will report information that may not be comparable.

One of the easiest methods for making a scale is to adapt the scale developed for measuring progress in general redesign projects (Milton et al. 1995) and shown in figure 4-1. Using this scale, the degree of component implementation is viewed as occurring in discrete steps that can be measured on a scale of zero to nine (10 steps). The 10 steps are used to measure the extent of progress for specific components, such as the use of acupressure or relaxation techniques or the inclusion of herbal preparations or homeopathic remedies on the initial intake or assessment form. This process allows the planning group to monitor the implementation of specific project components in many different areas of the organization. The wording of each

FIGURE 4-1. Scale for Determining Degree of Implementation

0	There is no current activity or planned action.
1	The idea is being explored.
2	There is an expressed commitment.
3	Discussions regarding participation are taking place.
4	A plan is developed.
5	Initial processes are implemented or piloted.
6	Processes are reviewed and refined.
7	There is a core of support for the component.
8	Most participants are implementing the component.
9	The component is an integral aspect of unit/department/ facility/system functioning.

Adapted, with permission, from D. Milton, J. Verran, R. Gerber, and J. Fleury. Tools to evaluate reengineering progress. In S. Blancett and D. Flarey, eds., *Reengineering Nursing and Health Care: The Handbook for Organizational Transformation* (Rockville, MD: Aspen Publishers, 1995). © 1995 Aspen Publishers, Inc.

step can be changed to incorporate the component being monitored. For example, step 3 can be changed from "Discussions regarding participation are taking place" to "Discussions regarding how staff will obtain information on admission about patient use of herbal preparations is taking place."

This scaling method allows an organization to measure progress not only of the integrative project in general, but also the specific components of the integration within the organization. For example, progress being made on a specific unit can be measured, as can integration of specific therapies in all the areas implementing them.

Step 6: Monitoring Staff Perceptions

In addition to measuring progress on how the specific components or elements of the project are being integrated, it is helpful to know if progress is also being made in how the project is being perceived. This is because most of the project components are implemented separately or sequentially, and staff may need frequent communication to remind them that the alternative and complementary therapies are part of a larger picture. The scaling method shown in figure 4-2, which can be used in a

FIGURE 4-2. Scale for Determining Staff Perceptions

1	People in the organization express a commitment to an integrative health care project.
2	The integrative health care project is described as the use of alternative and complementary therapies in addition to conventional care.
3	Some of the alternative and complementary therapies are seen as integrated with conventional care.
4	All of the alternative and complementary therapies are seen as integrated with conventional care.
5	The integrative health care project is seen as a unified model of alternative and complementary therapies and conventional care.

Adapted, with permission, from D. Milton, J. Verran, R. Gerber, and J. Fleury. Tools to evaluate reengineering progress. In S. Blancett and D. Flarey, eds., *Reengineering Nursing and Health Care: The Handbook for Organizational Transformation* (Rockville, MD: Aspen Publishers, 1995). © 1995 Aspen Publishers, Inc.

similar way to the scale for determining degree of implementation shown in figure 4-1, was developed for general redesign projects (Milton et al. 1995). It has been adapted to integrative health care project needs and can be used as is or modified to meet the needs of a specific organization.

Step 7: Developing Procedures for Collecting and Reviewing Information

Procedures for collecting essential monitoring information are needed. One person, most logically the project director, needs to assume responsibility for obtaining the data required for monitoring. If information is to be collected from several units or departments, then one person from each area is appointed both to collect information and make sure that it is sent to the project director. The project director has the task of compiling the information and providing reports to the planning group and the appropriate administrative staff. The planning group, with the input of administration as needed, has the critical job of reviewing the monitoring information and determining whether or not the project is on track. Regular monitoring permits the planning group to provide assistance to areas that are varying to a greater extent than planned.

Step 8: Determining Monitoring Frequency

It is important to determine how often monitoring is needed to see if what was planned is being implemented. Depending on the scope of the project, monthly or quarterly monitoring is probably appropriate. Frequent monitoring will assist in identifying which elements of the project are being implemented slowly or not at all, so that efforts to keep the project on track can be implemented early in the process. For example, if an organization finds that one clinical service or one group of providers is not implementing imagery to the extent that the other services or providers are, it is easier to explore why this is so and to provide necessary support in the earlier phases of the project, than to try to rectify the situation at the annual project evaluation.

Strategies to Reduce Conflict during Implementation

The most likely issue to arise during the implementation phase is opposition from those who do not want integrative health care. It is important for both the planning group and administration to realize that even if 10 years were devoted to planning, everyone would still not be pleased. Opposition to the project will come not only from those who do not want alternative therapies integrated with conventional care, but also from those who want the funds supporting the project to be used for other purposes. Patience and perseverance are required, and leaders must be strong enough to listen, yet withstand criticism and scrutiny.

Many strategies can help lessen the damage that can be done by conflict, including the following:

1. Integrating alternative therapies into existing programs
2. Involving selected resisters

3. Using administrative support
4. Educating the entire staff
5. Designing the initial phase as a research project
6. Involving outside leaders

It is important to remember throughout the duration of the project that even though these strategies can help, not all resistance or opposition can be eliminated. As with other projects, implementation of integrative health care cannot wait until all those who oppose it are avid supporters.

Strategy 1: Integrating Alternative Therapies into Existing Programs

Many organizations find that it is more difficult for the opposition if therapies are initially integrated within existing programs, rather than as a new program. For example, if guided imagery and acupuncture are integrated into an existing pain management program, they are woven into the fabric of services that already exist. Often, when therapies are integrated by providers who are already on staff and who are well-respected for their expertise in conventional care, there is a strong base for acceptance because the providers are already perceived as credentialed and qualified practitioners.

Strategy 2: Involving Selected Resisters

Another effective strategy is to involve opponents in the implementation process, including participation on committees that discuss the project, critique of research studies concerning alternative therapies, and attendance at integrative health care conferences with subsequent reports on the proceedings to the planning group or other groups in the organization.

For example, resisters can be involved in reviewing the research literature relevant to alternative therapies and integrative health care. They also can help to make sure that all are informed regarding the status of research in specific areas, updating that review, and making sure that copies of the research articles and critiques of them are available in the library. A special section of the library or a corner of a group practice can be devoted to these and other resources.

Involving the opposition has its dangers, however, and needs to be considered carefully, because those who resist a project can stymie activities and slow progress. It may be beneficial to understand that there are two different types of opposition: skeptics, who are open about their doubts but have a true commitment to people and high-quality care; and extremists, who personalize the issues, obstruct progress, and will most likely never be swayed. Skeptics may be of help and can, if convinced by evidence of integrative care's benefits, become strong allies and links to others. There is a danger in letting extremists participate on a committee because, generally speaking, obstructionism within the development team is very difficult to overcome and can unnecessarily hinder the project's chances of success.

Strategy 3: Using Administrative Support

There are many ways to show that the integrative health care project has the full support of administration, and this will clearly inform resisters that they will not be able to stop the project. There needs to be a senior administrator who both shares the vision of integrative care and has responsibility for the project, including an active role in all phases and most especially during implementation. This person ensures that the project remains consistent with the organizational culture and has the authority to make decisions that determine project success. One major function of the administrator is to empower the planning group—and then to buffer group members from those who continually oppose the project.

To insulate those who are responsible for implementation, it is necessary to have an independent budget for the project and, in some cases, even a separate company. Otherwise, integration efforts can become diluted with other organizational projects, and it can become difficult to release funds, even though the organization is committed to the project. For example, the integrative health care project will have a great need in the initial implementation phase for educational expenses such as programs, books, and tapes and for materials such as music and art that support an appropriate environment. From a financial perspective, it is very important to match the integrative health care project plan with available resources, and once those resources are allocated, they need to be protected to ensure project success.

The overall concern during this phase is for administration to provide continual support to those who are leading the effort so the vision does not get lost in the details of project implementation. It is easy when resistance to integrative health care arises to think the project is creating too much conflict and that it may be best to just abandon it. This is because the remainder of the organization's work needs to continue while this major change is occurring, and at times the rate and volume of change can seem overwhelming. It is at these times that the project director, planning group, and physician and/or nurse champions are most in need of an administrator's support and reminder of the importance of the project. This is not just one more project that needs to be done merely to satisfy accreditation requirements; the effort is being made so that people will have an array of options available to meet their health care needs. It cannot be overemphasized that, although there are certainly many strategies to increase the likelihood of project success, without a consistent vision and support of that vision by key organizational leaders, it is likely the project will fail regardless of the effort put forth.

Strategy 4: Educating the Entire Staff

Education of everyone involved in the project is a key strategy that helps all participants, including those who are resistant to integrative health care. Any organization that expects resistance (and that is the case with most systems) can begin the implementation phase of the project with education.

Some organizations have begun their efforts by stating that they are unsure whether or not they will ever integrate alternative and complementary therapies into conventional care at their facilities. However, because the people who use their services and the people in the community they serve are using these therapies, providers and staff need to be knowledgeable about these modalities and types of care. The premise is that people want to ask questions about all aspects of their health care, not just conventional care, and it is best if the health care professionals in the organization can answer all of these questions.

Many organizations also realize that they need to include questions for obtaining information about the use of alternative and complementary therapies on assessment or intake forms. Educating providers about these therapies, ways of asking about therapies people commonly use, and how to answer the questions people frequently ask about their use can be less threatening ways to begin implementation, as well as providing helpful information to both staff and patients.

Strategy 5: Designing the Initial Phase as a Research Project

Another strategy that helps to reduce resistance in the beginning of implementation is to design the initial phase as a research or demonstration project. This might be a six-month demonstration project to determine the extent to which integration of alternative therapies achieves specific outcomes. For example, the initial phase of integration could be the introduction of the use of Therapeutic Touch on an oncology unit to care for people with pain management problems. A project evaluation could be designed to examine the change, if any, in pain management and patient satisfaction after integration of the new therapy. An evaluation introduces the perspective of objectivity; the organization can introduce integration of alternative therapies thereafter with less opposition. If the introduction of these therapies is not effective in improving outcomes, the project can be redesigned or discontinued. It can be beneficial to include those who oppose or are resistant to integrative care in the group that is responsible for the project evaluation.

Designing the initial phase as a research project also may encourage students in the organization to help with some aspects of project design or evaluation and use that experience to meet school requirements. Students are frequently required to conduct literature reviews or project evaluations; having materials available can make integrative health care more appealing to students as a topic. Employees who are graduate students can help to compile an extensive reference list, much of which needs to be evidence-based if possible, which can be reviewed by those who are skeptical regarding the integration of alternative therapies.

Strategy 6: Involving Outside Leaders

Whether or not the opposition to integrative health care is from those within the organization or from members of the community, it can be helpful to bring outsiders into the organization and for the organization to take its message to the community and the national level. Presentations given by outside experts in the selected alternative therapies or by others who are knowledgeable in answering questions about a variety of alternative therapies can be helpful. Practitioners and administrators can gain added support for their vision by inviting those who have experience in integrative health care projects to present at inservices or grand rounds. Many times advice from presenters or consultants is considered to be of considerable value because these experts, authors or experts staff members have met at conferences or meetings, come from outside the organization and are more objective. An overview of some organizations or groups that are integrating alternative therapies into conventional care, as well as key leaders within those organizations or groups, is provided in appendix B.

Involvement in the local and national community is valuable during the implementation process. If the local community is kept informed regarding what is actually being implemented in the organization, it can eliminate the upset that can happen when people hear only part of the plan and do not know just what is being offered. Administrators and practitioners need to keep the board of directors, advisory board, local community, and professional groups, as well as local and national regulatory agencies, aware of the organization's plan and implementation activities. Key community and professional organization leaders are invaluable in this process; it is important to remember that two-way communication with these leaders can help eliminate or at least reduce opposition from within and outside the organization.

Effective Communication

One of the themes that underlies much of the implementation phase is the need for continual, two-way communication. It is the responsibility of administration, the project director, and the planning group to make sure that the communication activities that were planned actually occur. Copies of minutes and periodic project reports need to be sent to those on the distribution list. Phone calls to key community and organization leaders, as well as to those on the board of directors and advisory board, keep lines of communication open. Many organizations find that use of computer technology is especially helpful and cost-effective. Internet chat and discussion rooms can be used for raising issues that develop during implementation and allow for quick response. Also, much education can be done on-line. For example, practitioners can benefit from a case presentation placed on-line each week wherein each discipline can respond to the clinical problems of the patient from its unique, yet interrelated perspective. Everyone has the opportunity to contribute input about which alternative and conventional therapies they would integrate to help in providing care, and to learn about the practical aspects of integrating care from each other. Again, the project director needs to make sure that someone is responsible for coordinating the on-line communication and forwarding any problems or issues that arise to the planning group. Analysis of on-line communication can be an excellent source of ideas for practitioner education and a way to uncover practical concerns when developing protocols, policies, and procedures.

A good way to make sure that people remain informed even if they are unable to attend meetings is to record proceedings and make copies of slides and notes from presentations for those who are unable to attend. Busy staff rarely attend all meetings and, although meeting minutes can help, especially if they are brief and concise, a video or cassette tape is usually more interesting. People who cannot attend in person can often be present via teleconferencing or can participate in a closed discussion room on-line. This is always helpful for staff and committee members because they can use virtual time to tune in and express opinions, which keeps them active as participants.

Subscribing to peer-reviewed journals in alternative therapies or integrative care can continue to inspire interest and keep
members informed regarding what is occurring at other organizations. Forwarding copies of key references or articles to planning group members helps to maintain involvement as well.

Conclusion

Implementation of integrative health care will occur at different
rates throughout the organization, and overall progress as well
as the degree of implementation in each department needs to
be monitored throughout this phase. The extent to which people in the organization view the project as a change in philosophy, rather than just the integration of selected alternative
and complementary therapies, needs to be monitored as well.
Various strategies can be used to prevent or at least reduce the
impact of issues that can arise during implementation, but the
importance of maintaining the overall project vision and open
communication is crucial. The next chapter describes the evaluation process and discusses issues that influence project evaluation design.

Reference Cited

Milton, D., J. Verran, R. Gerber, and J. Fleury. 1995. Tools to
evaluate reengineering progress. In *Reengineering Nursing
and Health Care: The Handbook for Organizational Transformation*, S. Blancett and D. Flarey, eds. Rockville, MD: Aspen.

5

Evaluating Integrative Health Care

E valuation of outcomes can help health care providers and consumers identify positive or negative variations in practice, measure and control costs, and assess the impact of new technologies (Bootman 1998). Evaluation projects that show the effectiveness of interventions may be especially useful for providers of alternative therapies.

The focus of this chapter is on the evaluation phase of the integrative health care project. Within the three basic steps of design, data collection, and data analysis and interpretation, are suggestions for selecting outcome measures, determining appropriate data collection tools, and ensuring the validity and reliability of data. There are many resources that may be consulted for detailed information on each step in the evaluation process. This chapter gives a basic overview of the process and highlights special considerations for integrative care projects.

The steps outlined in this chapter adhere as closely as possible to conventional evaluation methods, and this adherence is important for two reasons. The first is that reports on integrative care projects are closely scrutinized by the conventional community; when flaws in methodology are noted, the results may be discounted. The second reason is that those who believe in integrative health care have a responsibility to use evaluation methods that will promote the development of valid and reliable projects and interventions.

Step 1: Design

Although there is considerable evidence of the popularity of alternative therapies with consumers, many in the scientific community remain unconvinced of their effectiveness. In part, this skepticism results from the methodological flaws present in many reports related to alternative therapies. For results to be useful to both the organization performing the evaluation and the health care field as a whole, the evaluation process must be well planned to avoid methodological errors. The overall design of the process comprises the approach to be used, the population to be addressed, the outcomes to be measured, and the early identification of variables that may skew results.

Selecting an Approach

Investigational approaches fall into three basic categories: descriptive, correlational, and experimental and quasi-experimental.

- The *descriptive approach* allows researchers to determine the level of something, such as the level of patient satisfaction regarding pain management, or to identify an array of factors that affect a specific outcome, such as the factors influencing people's choice of acupuncture instead of a conventional care option.
- A *correlational approach* allows researchers to determine any associations between factors that may be important to a specific outcome. For example, if community members express satisfaction with an organization's provision of alternative therapies, this response may be related to one or more community-specific demographics (age, income level, race, and so on).
- *Experimental* and *quasi-experimental* *approaches* allow researchers to determine the effectiveness of specific alternative therapies or of an entire integrative health care program. For example, an experimental design may evaluate whether people are better able to manage their pain after being taught relaxation techniques. Most intervention studies

that compare or contrast the effect of conventional care versus integrative care on outcomes use quasi-experimental designs. For example, many well-controlled trials demonstrate the effectiveness of acupuncture for low back pain (Coan et al. 1980; Fox and Melzack 1976; Gunn et al. 1980; Laitenen 1976; MacDonald et al. 1983).

All of these approaches are quantitative in nature, meaning they involve collection of data using specific and objective measures. (Outcome measures and types of data are discussed later in this chapter.) Qualitative approaches that can provide information regarding people's perceptions of the care experience also may be used. For example, a qualitative study may focus on what having a wide array of care options means to people or on what people's first experiences of acupuncture are like.

Some projects are best evaluated using either a quantitative or a qualitative approach; others may employ both methods. Quantitative measurement collects data in certain predetermined categories (Patton 1980) and is useful for showing how a situation has changed. For example, a quantitative methodology may be used to show whether a program aimed at reducing acute asthma attacks resulted in an increased, decreased, or unchanged occurrence rate. The advantage in using quantitative methods is that they furnish clear, understandable information, and it takes relatively little time to collect data. The disadvantage of this approach is that researchers cannot tell what factors accounted for the results shown. For example, a study that measured the number of asthma attack occurrences would not provide information about factors such as people's sense of control or environmental conditions that might trigger attacks.

Qualitative methods supply more complex data through the use of open-ended questions or observations. For instance, asking people what they found most helpful about a guided imagery session might provide a variety of answers. These answers may differ from what the care provider intended, but the patients' responses would be important to include in any judgments made about the program. Qualitative methods are time-consuming, but can enrich the information available for use in decision making.

Selecting an Appropriate Population

The population to be used in the evaluation will influence the design of the project in a number of ways. If the focus population is a group with similar characteristics (called *homogenous*), the methods for collecting information may differ than if the focus population is diverse (*heterogeneous*). For example, the evaluation process would differ if the goal were to evaluate treatments for women between the ages of 30 and 50 with cluster headaches (homogenous group), than if the focus were to examine the health-related quality of life for all people receiving homeopathic treatment (heterogeneous group). Defining the target population in the most specific way possible provides an explicit focus for the evaluation.

Certainly, collecting information from every patient or community member involved in the project would provide the most valid results. However, efforts of this magnitude are seldom feasible in terms of time and cost. As a result, most integrative health care projects collect information from a sample of the overall population. Even though evaluation projects usually sample from a population that is convenient and readily available, care must be taken in selecting a sample that is representative of the overall group.

Representativeness and Recruitment of Participants

The issue of representativeness is a key to all phases of project evaluation. Representativeness refers to the degree to which the qualities of the sample reflect those of the whole group. For example, in conducting a survey to assess community satisfaction with a new integrative pain management program, it is important to make sure that respondents are chosen from across all demographic groups (age, gender, race, ethnicity, income level, and so on).

Recruitment of people who will be used in evaluations of integrative care is a major concern. Those who seek integrative services may be a skewed population and more likely than would a general population to respond positively to alternative therapies. This difficulty can be lessened by recruiting subjects from the population with the given medical condition or by working closely with insurance companies to identify a population for evaluation of care.

Sample Size

A frequently discussed topic regarding sample population is that of size. In determining sample, investigators frequently have to balance the need to collect data efficiently and the desire to have a statistically powerful result. Scientific methods exist for determining sample size based on estimates of the effect or potency of the treatment, the level of significance selected for the project, and the data analysis technique used. This method is referred to as *power analysis*, and readers interested in more information regarding this technique are referred to the work of Cohen (1988). However, convention suggests that a sample size of at least 30 subjects in each comparison group can provide useful data. Thirty subjects also are necessary for the commonly used data analysis programs, such as the Statistical Package for the Social Sciences (SPSS-PC+). (Data analysis is discussed later in this chapter.)

Although collecting data from a very large sample may be attractive because of the corresponding ability to detect subtle differences in outcomes for treatment groups, the cost of such an effort may be prohibitive to a group practice or solo provider. If this type of sample is specifically desired, however, it may be helpful to join forces with an existing academic or clinical data collection project.

Selecting Outcome Measures

The project objectives for the evaluation phase are the same as those identified in the planning stage. These objectives are used to help determine the purpose of the evaluation and the outcome measures used. Outcome measures can address program objectives that relate to overall program results, such as costs, community satisfaction with care, or market share, or they can relate to outcomes of care for people with clinical conditions or symptoms. These patient-related measures include health status outcomes such as quality of life and pain management.

Table 5-1 shows the most common categories of outcomes to be evaluated and examples of measures used for each.

A variety of generic measures are available that can help assess the overall effects of either alternative therapy interventions or integrative health care programs. The outcome measures with which clinicians are most familiar involve changes in health status, such as physiological states, functioning, and affective states. Traditionally, investigators have used rates of morbidity and mortality as well as utilization of health care services to indicate health status. However, morbidity/mortality rates are very rough measures of health outcomes and have limited value when examining the effects of specific alternative therapies or integrative protocols. In addition, traditional measures do not reflect patients' perceptions of health status. The following discussion provides descriptions of a number of commonly used generic health status measures that providers of alternative therapies may want to consider as part of an evaluation plan.

Health-Related Quality of Life

Instruments used to measure health-related quality of life (HRQOL) most often provide very broad definitions of well-being. The concepts included in HRQOL instruments are those

TABLE 5-1. Measures Selected for Specific Types of Outcomes

Types of Outcomes	Examples of Measures
Biological or physiological factors	Blood pressure, cholesterol level
	Morbidity, mortality
Social and psychological factors	Perception of symptoms
	Perception of health-related quality of life
Environmental/economic factors	Hospitalizations, emergency department visits
	Expenses for medications
Functional health status measures	Satisfaction with care
	Return to work status

related to perceptions of impairments, functional status, social and emotional roles, and expectations about the duration of life (Patrick and Deyo 1989). Each instrument defines these components somewhat differently, and the definitions must be examined closely by those who intend to use the instruments. In addition to the definitions of health, issues to consider when selecting an HRQOL instrument include the clinical relevance of the information derived from the instrument, as well as the reliability and validity of the population of interest. (The concepts of reliability and validity are discussed later in this chapter.)

Originally developed by the Rand Corporation, one of the most commonly used HRQOL instruments, the Short Form-36, also called the SF-36 (Ware and Sherbourne 1992), is used with people across the continuum of health status. The SF-36 provides information about health status related to eight areas of functioning and well-being. Investigators suggest that it is most relevant for a generally healthy population. Indeed, one of the criticisms is that it is not sensitive enough to detect changes among those already experiencing incapacity. Advantages to the SF-36 include its wide use and recognition, the ease of administration and scoring, and a sampling from a broad range of health status indicators. Also, many organizations and group practices use the SF-36, so it is often used for comparison purposes across groups of people and facilities and for benchmarking. Other instruments that are used to assess HRQOL include the Sickness Impact Profile (Bergner et al. 1976), the Nottingham Health Profile (Hunt et al. 1980), and the Duke Health Profile (Parkerson et al. 1990).

Patient Satisfaction with Care

Satisfaction with care may be one area in which providers of alternative therapies would find especially useful information. Satisfaction is derived from many perspectives and includes patient expectations of care, the outcomes of care, and emotional and cognitive components of satisfaction. Patient satisfaction with care has been closely linked to patients' assessment of the quality of care received (Hall et al. 1993) and to compliance with the treatment regimen.

Satisfaction can influence patients' decisions to terminate relationships with physicians/providers. As the competition to attract health care consumers becomes more intense, the desire to demonstrate satisfaction with care takes on increasing importance to providers. Providers of integrative care often want to see if there is any difference in patient satisfaction when alternative therapies are integrated with conventional care.

Considerations for Patient Satisfaction Measures   The dimensions of satisfaction with care encompass judgments about a variety of factors, including technical quality of care, interpersonal aspects of care, access, and convenience, as well as overall satisfaction (Ware and Hays 1988). Most satisfaction instruments, however, seldom incorporate all aspects. The most frequently used instrument for obtaining patient satisfaction data is the survey, and a wide variety of satisfaction surveys are available. The usefulness of the data produced by them hinges on several factors, which include the method of sampling, the method of administration, and concerns related to measurement error. These factors are addressed elsewhere in this chapter. The main concern in measuring patient satisfaction is that the instrument used contain items to which people respond differently if integrative care is having the desired impact.

When patient satisfaction surveys are incorporated into an evaluation plan, the survey results need to be evaluated carefully. Item descriptions need to allow the reviewer to determine what factors of care are sampled, as well as the likelihood of generating socially desirable responses. In addition, the description of survey methods needs to list the steps taken to decrease measurement error. Judgments about these issues can guide providers to surveys that provide relevant information.

Visual Analogue Scales

A variety of condition-specific measuring devices exist. One of the most commonly used is the Visual Analogue Scale (VAS), which consists of a 100-mm-long straight line, oriented either vertically or horizontally, with the ends identified as opposite response to subjective experience. For example, if the VAS were used to assess pain intensity, the ends, or anchors, of the line would be labeled "no pain at all" and "most intense pain that can be imagined." Subjects place a mark on the line to indicate their assessment of the experience in question. The VAS is an attractive choice in evaluations related to subjective experiences because it provides ratio-level data that can be used with powerful statistical techniques such as t tests or analysis of variance.

Visual Analogue Scales have been demonstrated to be reliable and valid in the measurement of a number of subjective topics including experimental pain (Price et al. 1983), clinical pain following hip arthroplasty (deNies and Fidler 1997), anxiety related to gastrointestinal endoscopic procedures (Bampton and Draper 1997), mood changes related to sleep deprivation (Dinges et al. 1997), dyspnea in people with chronic obstructive pulmonary disease (Mishima et al. 1996), and feelings of hunger and fullness (Gielkens et al. 1998). Further, the VAS has demonstrated sensitivity in distinguishing pain intensity and pain unpleasantness (Price and Harkins 1987). (One drawback is that a small portion of subjects have difficulty conceptualizing their experiences on a straight line.) Because it is easy to use and the results are easily interpreted, the VAS can be used with confidence as a measure of subjective phenomena. In evaluating integrative care, it can be used to determine the effects of either a single alternative therapy or to determine any differences in outcomes between integrative and conventional care.

Planning for Variation

One helpful activity in the design phase of evaluation projects is to explore the variety of factors that could influence why, how, when, where, and for whom an alternative therapy or integrative care protocol will have the desired outcome. These factors may be classified as contextual (environmental) or confounding (related to patient condition). In order to make meaningful comparisons regarding outcomes, it is necessary to adjust for differences that result from types and severity of conditions that people experience. Judgments about the results of care can be made only when characteristics such as patient age, diagnosis, and comorbidity factors (for example, diabetes or cardiovascular conditions) are addressed. Risk adjustment is especially important for nonexperimental investigations, because the procedures commonly employed to overcome bias in experimental designs may not be available.

Severity refers to the extent of the condition or the effects of the illness on the patient, while comorbidity refers to the potential results of the presence of additional clinical factors such as heart disease, renal failure, and others (Kane 1997). It is important to compare individuals with similar pretreatment conditions when making judgments about the effects of health care interventions. For example, acupuncture may appear to decrease low back pain more than does conventional care, but the comparison is not valid if one group had previous back surgery and the other group did not.

Another variable that may be important in the evaluation of alternative therapies is the method of delivery of services. Many who practice alternative therapies contend that elements of the relationship between the receiver and the provider of care play an important role in the outcome of treatment. In order to obtain an appropriate evaluation of alternative therapies, the influence of the care provider must be taken into account. That is, some evaluation reports of the effectiveness of a specific alternative therapy such as homeopathy, for example, may not be an evaluation of homeopathy as much as they are evaluations of the relationship between the provider and patients. A strategy to help deal with this concern is to use patients of several homeopathic practitioners.

Step 2: Data Collection

Data collection requires more time and attention than any other portion of the project. Because of the expense associated with collection activities, the time it takes to select a methodology that will produce consistent and accurate data is worth the effort. Several factors regarding the type of data to be collected and the tools and methods to be used need to be addressed at this step.

Choosing an Appropriate Level of Data

Information may be gathered at a variety of levels; individual, group, and organization are the most common. There is no one best level for analysis; rather, the reason for evaluation often dictates the level of data to be collected and analyzed. Many researchers suggest that including information from multiple levels gives a broader and more complete perspective on evaluation activities (Rousseau 1985).

Individual-Level Data

Most clinicians are familiar with data that have been collected from and about individuals. Examples of data collected at the individual level include evaluations of the effectiveness of homeopathic remedies for chronic pain and assessment of the effects of Therapeutic Touch on wound healing. Most patient satisfaction surveys represent data collected at the individual level; that is, all of the statements to which people are asked to respond are focused on the experience of one individual's experiences or ratings.

Individual-level responses are used for analysis of mean values and comparisons between groups of people. Because most readily available data collection instruments address individuals, and clinicians can easily identify the usefulness of this type of data, the use of this level of data can be advantageous. The disadvantage is that it may not provide the information that an organization needs. For example, an organization may not get an accurate read on how supportive a department is concerning integrating alternative therapies solely by asking some individuals in that department how they feel about the possibility. Individual-level data are very helpful in providing data about the experiences of individuals, but not of groups.

Group-Level Data

Group-level data are often used to analyze the effect of care delivered by a group of providers or a group's perceptions of an experience. Patients' rates of complications after specific surgical procedures is an example of group-level data; the rate of complications cannot be attributed to any one person or department. An examination of the effects of introducing integrative health care on a group's cohesion is another example. Perceptions of group cohesion reflect how well the group is functioning collectively.

The advantage of using group-level data is that most processes of care are accomplished by a group of caregivers, and often what investigators truly want to examine is the result of that group's efforts. The disadvantage is that it is not measured frequently, so few instruments have been developed with the group as the unit of analysis. In addition, special care needs to be taken in choosing or defining an instrument intended to measure group-level data so that the measure is valid and reliable.

Organization-Level Data

Many clinicians are more familiar with organization-level data than with group-level data. Examples include average length of stay, total charges, and patient satisfaction with care. Advantages of including these data in evaluation are that they are easily understood and easy to gather; most health care facilities have financial and resource utilization systems that produce organization-level data. One problem in using this level of data is that it is not sensitive to subtle changes. For example, implementation of alternative therapies for one group of patients may not produce effects on patient satisfaction surveys. However, an evaluation that draws from a variety of levels of measurement will provide stronger evidence and be more useful for decision making.

Establishing a Time Frame

An important part of the data collection strategy includes decisions about the time frame for collection activities. The most commonly used time frames involve either retrospective or prospective data collection. Retrospective data collection looks back at events that have already occurred, whereas a prospective strategy involves collecting data as it happens or right after it has happened. Retrospective data collection often relies on documentation and is frequently hampered by inadequate charting or documentation of the specific alternative therapy or protocol that was used. This method rarely includes needed information about other factors that influenced the outcome. If the project focuses on retrospective data, making sure that essential data elements are included consistently in the records saves time and frustration. Data collected in a way that does not rely on documentation may be more reliable than traditional methods. For example, having people rate their back pain at specific intervals following acupuncture treatment may be more useful than relying on the pain level after acupuncture as documented in the patients' records.

Prospective data collection can sometimes be affected by caregivers' awareness of what is being studied. An example of this type of effect is that pain ratings may improve after acupuncture treatments because a practitioner is aware that someone will be examining the documentation. Practitioners may emphasize the pain relief that can be expected without consciously exhibiting bias.

Selecting Data Collection Instruments

The purpose of the evaluation project, the outcomes to be studied, the measures to be used, and the types of data to be collected all influence what instrument(s) will be employed for data collection. The factors to consider when choosing an appropriate instrument include its reliability and validity and whether an established tool can be used or a new one must be created.

Desirable Characteristics

The two major characteristics with which investigators should be concerned when selecting an instrument are validity and reliability. These characteristics are also important for selecting outcome measures, as mentioned earlier in the chapter. Because of the strong link between the outcomes selected and the data collection instrument used to measure them, they are examined together here.

Validity   Validity is the degree to which an instrument or process describes or is consistent with the concept it is supposed to measure. For example, an instrument or survey that claims to measure patient satisfaction or degree of pain is valid to the extent that it measures those concepts. Validity is not assessed in absolute terms, but rather within the context of its use. For example, measures of restlessness may be valid with a group of people suffering acute pain, but inappropriate and invalid for people with dementia.

Attention needs to be given to the validity of the outcome chosen for review as well as to the intervention selected for evaluation. In terms of the outcome of interest, there has to be a logical connection between the outcome and/or process of care and the measures selected to represent the results. Because data collection is time consuming, it is important to make sure that clear and logical links exist between the intervention or process change and the outcome of care. An example may be drawn from information about patient education. Although it is clear that patient education is a useful and necessary part of treatment, care needs to be taken in linking the educational intervention to patient outcomes. It is reasonable to evaluate patient education in terms of resulting knowledge, but it may not be valid to link educational sessions to changes in behavior.

By way of illustration, the fact that many people know about the effect of obesity on hypertension does not mean that everyone who is hypertensive undertakes a weight loss diet. In this instance, if individual weight loss were selected as the outcome of the evaluation project, patient education may not be a valid intervention to associate with the selected outcome. Outcome categories most frequently examined include physiologic measures, functional status, satisfaction, or absence of complications. Issues such as severity of illness and comorbidities may have such a profound impact on patients' outcomes that the whole investigation may yield misleading (and invalid) results if these are not taken into account.

Reliability   Reliability refers to the degree to which an instrument or tool can be depended on to give consistent results. For example, a provider rating of degree of pain relief is reliable to the extent that all providers who see people with the same level of pain would give the patients the same scores. The importance of reliability in the data collection process cannot be overemphasized because the applicability of the results hinge on the consistency of the data collection instruments and methods. Two issues to consider when thinking about reliability are stability and equivalence.

Stability refers to the consistency of repeated uses or measures. This is easily illustrated by use of hand temperature to measure state of relaxation. If the instrument used to measure hand temperature indicated the temperature as 80° F at one time, but 68° F a few minutes later with no significant change in circumstances, that instrument would not be considered to be very stable and, therefore, not reliable.

Equivalence may be defined as the assurance that two methods, individuals, or data collection tools yield very similar results. An example of equivalence would be a comparison of two observers rating range of motion. If the observers failed to agree in their ratings to a great extent (> 90 percent), they would not be considered equivalent; therefore, the method would be unreliable.

Types of Instruments

The type and quality of data collection instruments can affect the reliability of information obtained. The choice of measurement instruments most often is a reflection of the objectives of the project. For example, if the integrative health care project was designed to improve patient functional status, then an instrument such as the SF-36 (Ware and Sherbourne 1992) would likely be used. Other techniques frequently used in data collection include interviews with individuals or focus groups, observations, and surveys or questionnaires. One can either use an established instrument or create a new one for the program evaluation or study.

Established Instruments   Using established or published instruments for investigations of alternative therapies strengthens the design of studies because they have been tested scientifically and have demonstrated reliability and validity. Development and testing of a new instrument is a long and burdensome task, which often takes several years. In addition, if certain parameters are met, results can be compared to the results of other investigations in which the same instrument was used. Questions to consider before using a published instrument include the following:

- What was the purpose for which it was developed?
- What was the target population for which it was originally designed?
- Did it specify an age group, gender, or disease entity?
- For what setting was the original instrument designed?

- How were the concepts included in it defined?
- How do the purpose, population, setting, and concepts for the current project compare to those for which the instrument was designed?
- Is there sufficient evidence of its reliability?
- Is there information about its validity?
- Is the instrument able to be read and comprehended by the group included in this project?
- What sort of demands will be placed on the study subjects in terms of completing the instrument?
- Are there any risks to the subjects that could result from its administration?
- Is there information available that describes how to obtain it?
- Is there information available about how to administer and score it?

One disadvantage of using an established instrument is that the concepts represented in the published instrument may not match those in the present project. The large number of instruments that measure health-related quality of life offer a good example of the variety of ways in which a concept can be defined. Another disadvantage is the fee charged for its use.

New Instruments   If no established instrument exists that appropriately measures the outcome, project evaluators may consider designing a new instrument. When developing a data collection instrument, there are several ways to improve the usefulness and relevance of the information it produces, including use of a panel of experts and careful construction of the survey/questionnaire/observation items.

A group of experts familiar with the clinical or practice area and the alternative therapies being integrated can offer comments on the clarity, completeness, and usefulness of the instrument items. In addition, these experts can suggest necessary changes to the items or the format of the items. This authoritative review strengthens the data collection tool and lends credibility to the data collection process.

When constructing surveys, questionnaires, or observation checklists, each item needs to be examined for its ability to produce data related to a single portion of the evaluation. Items that are short and ask about a single behavior or observation are more likely to provide usable results. Information that is not essential but would be "good to have" should be avoided. Each item needs to be clearly stated and unambiguous. For example, an observation checklist item that states "Patient able to button shirt and fasten pants" would be better stated if written as two separate items.

Implementing Data Collection

Strategies for collecting data involve determining what the end product should look like as well as how it will be analyzed. For example, if investigators want to be able to describe the age, gender, marital status, functional status, and length of stay of patients receiving a particular alternative therapy, data collection might include medical record review, administration of a patient questionnaire, and retrieval of financial information. Concerns about the validity and reliability of data collected require consideration of both the method of administration for data collection and the possibility of measurement error.

Method of Administration

The method of survey administration needs to be chosen to ensure that responses reflect what people really think or feel about their care, rather than what is socially desirable. The temptation to give answers that one believes the surveyor wants is evident in the overwhelming positive approval that almost all satisfaction surveys report (Carr-Hill 1992). Methods that ensure confidentiality as well as precision in question construction can improve the usefulness of survey results. Also, it is best to remember that the patients who are most likely to complete satisfaction surveys are those who are very satisfied or very dissatisfied with care. This lack of variation in response creates difficulties in evaluation.

Measurement Error

A concern inherent in all types of surveys is the degree of measurement error introduced by the process. All instruments and methods of evaluation contain measurement error, but the prudent researcher takes steps to reduce it whenever possible. Measurement error can be introduced into survey results in the way the survey is conducted or administered, by the design of the questions, and through characteristics of those who respond. Interviews that are conducted by telephone or face-to-face can produce different results than the same questions on a written questionnaire mailed back to the organization anonymously.

In addition, the time frame in which the survey is administered influences responses. For example, different results will be obtained if satisfaction is measured immediately after an encounter with a care provider than if the survey is given four to six weeks following treatment. The construction and ordering of survey items also influence the response to the items. Survey items that are designed to address only one aspect of care are helpful. However, even well-constructed items can be presented in such a way that the responder tends to pick a particular response category and answer all questions in the same way. This tendency is referred to as response-set bias and is frequently encountered in survey research. Those using information from satisfaction surveys need to examine the results to determine the extent of response set.

Training Staff

Regardless of the type of data collection instrument used, those who are to gather data need to be trained and monitored to ensure data reliability. Training most frequently takes the form of describing the aim of the activity, discussing the definition of terms, and explaining the response alternatives. In addition, it is useful to conduct some comparison of data collectors' responses to the same events or items. For example, by asking two or three care providers to use the same instrument to evaluate the same patient's performance of a task, it would be possible to determine to what degree the observers' responses are comparable. In this way, one can be more certain that the differences seen in the results were really due to the differences in patients' conditions, rather than to differences in the observers' judgments.

Step 3: Data Analysis

Data analysis involves organizing and handling data so that they have some meaning. Procedures used to analyze data correspond to the different types of evaluation designs. That is, descriptive analysis is used to describe a population used or the information obtained, correlational analysis is used to determine associations among factors, and experimental analysis is used to determine the outcomes of therapies or programs.

Descriptive Analysis

Commonly used analysis techniques involve descriptions and comparisons of the data or groups and may include comparisons across time. In terms of descriptive statistics, statistical tests most frequently used are those that produce the mean, range, standard deviation, and frequencies of occurrences. Percentages of items may also be included in descriptive analysis techniques. Measures such as the mean, range, and standard deviation (also called measures of central tendency) provide information about the variability of the data. These measures have meaning when the item being examined is measured on a scale or as a rating, but are not appropriate when the item is a category, such as type of diagnosis or gender.

Correlational Analysis

When examining relationships among factors, correlational procedures are appropriate. For example, correlational data analysis would be used to examine the relationship between job conflict and the incidence of low back pain. The results inform us about the association between the two variables; for example, the results will tell whether or not job conflict and low back pain are related, but not whether the low back pain is caused by job conflict. Correlational analyses are helpful if little is known in the area and it would be difficult or premature to set up an evaluation project with a sophisticated experimental design. Pearson's product moment and Kendall's tau seem to be the most frequently used correlational techniques.

Experimental Analysis

When examining comparisons of data over time or by group, t test and analysis of variance (ANOVA) are the techniques most frequently used. A variety of computer programs such as Excel and SPSS can prove very useful with data analysis. Statistical techniques such as the t test or ANOVA can be appropriately used when comparing two groups or the same group at two different times. These techniques may be used when the data have a discrete value or are measured as a scale or rating. Both the t test and ANOVA produce a result called an F value and a significance level, or p value. Level of significance refers to the probability that the results could have been arrived at by chance. Many times a p value of .05 is chosen, which indicates that the probability of the result happening by chance is 5 out of 100. The investigator determines the level of significance before starting data analysis procedures. When interpreting the results, if the p value does not reach the predetermined point, the F value is meaningless, since the two groups do not show significant difference on that item. If, however, the p value is appropriate, the F value indicates the degree of difference between groups.

Many evaluation issues are no different from those that are encountered in evaluation of outcomes in allopathic care. For example, many allopathic interventions can be tried for patients with asthma, yet it is difficult to identify which intervention was responsible for improvement in the condition. It is also possible that none of the interventions used had an actual effect; positive outcomes in the patient's condition may have been the result solely of being seen more frequently by health care providers. Outcomes such as decreased frequency of emergency room visits, dependence on prescription medications, and perceived shortness of breath may improve regardless of interventions used. One technique that can be used to get around this is to establish a degree of response that could not be expected solely because of placebo response or the effect of being seen frequently. For example, an FEV-1 on pulmonary function tests that shows a statistically significant improvement of 15 percent or greater would clearly not have been the result of placebo.

Conclusion

This chapter provides an extensive overview of the issues that need to be considered in evaluation and describes many strategies that can be used. However, it is key to any project or care evaluation to have access to the services of an evaluation methodologist and statistician. Many physicians, other health care professionals, and administrators are not expert in these areas, and if expert consultation is not sought, often the appropriate data are not collected and the results are of no value in decision making. And, unless the information obtained can be used to make a decision regarding project progress or outcome, or the value of specific interventions integrated into conventional care, it is irrelevant how sophisticated the evaluation design was.

If these services are not available in an organization or group practice, many expert methodologists are mentioned in research and evaluation articles, or university faculty with expertise in this area might be helpful. Research institutions are well equipped to provide these services, but their focus on basic science research and use of the randomized controlled trial in a blinded, placebo-controlled study may be unsuitable. Examining the effects of alternative therapies in clinical trials in smaller institutions may be difficult if conventional evaluation measures cannot be used because treatments are individualized. The challenge in evaluating these therapies is to explore creative, valid evaluation methodologies. For example, perhaps acupuncture can be studied using sham acupuncture points, or Therapeutic Touch can be studied using a mock form of the process.

It is difficult, as well, to obtain funding for the evaluation of integrative health care. There is little financial benefit for private industry to finance the needed research because the technologies are not patentable. Herbs and acupuncture, for example, are not patentable; they remain within the public domain. Single-remedy homeopathic remedies are not patentable and as such attract little or no private investment in research. Most evaluation of integrative health care, whether that evaluation focuses on general organizational outcomes or specific health status-related measures, will come from the integration of evaluation principles into conventional care settings that provide integrative care.

References Cited

Bampton, P., and B. Draper. 1997. Effect of relaxation music on patient tolerance of gastrointestinal endoscopic procedures. *Journal of Clinical Gastroenterology* 25 (1): 343–45.

Bergner, M., R. Bobbitt, S. Kressel, W. Pollard, B. Gilson, and J. Morris. 1976. The Sickness Impact Profile: Conceptual formulation and methodological development of a health status index. *International Journal of Health Services* 6: 393.

Bootman, J. L. 1998. Keynote address. Arizona Health Outcomes Research Conference. March 27, Phoenix.

Carr-Hill, R. A. 1992. The measurement of patient satisfaction. *Journal of Public Health Medicine* 14 (3): 236–49.

Coan, R., G. Wong, S. L. Ku, et al. 1980. The acupuncture treatment of low back pain: A randomized controlled treatment. *American Journal of Chinese Medicine* 8: 181.

Cohen, J. 1988. *Statistical Power Analysis for the Behavioral Sciences*. 2d ed. Hillsdale, NJ: Lawrence Erlbaum Associates.

DeNies, F., and M. W. Fidler. 1997. Visual analog scale for the assessment of total hip arthroplasty. *Journal of Arthroplasty* 12 (4): 416–19.

Dinges, D. F., F. Pack, K. Williams, K. A. Gillen, J. W. Powell, G. E. Ott, C. Aptowicz, and A. I. Pack. 1997. Cumulative sleepiness, mood disturbance and psychomotor vigilance performance decrements during a week of sleep restricted to 4-5 hours per night. *Sleep* 20 (4): 267–70.

Fox, E., and R. Melzack. 1976. Transcutaneous stimulation and acupuncture: Comparison of treatment for low back pain. *Pain* 2: 141.

Gielkens, H. A. J., M. Verkijk, W. F. Lam, C. B. H. W. Lamers, and A. A. M. Masclee. 1998. Effects of hyperglycemia and hyperinsulinemia on satiety in humans. *Metabolism* 47 (3): 321–24.

Gunn, C. C., W. E. Milbrandt, A. S. Little, et al. 1980. Dry needling of muscle motor points for chronic low back pain. *Spine* 5 (3): 279.

Hall, J. A., M. A. Milburn, and A. M. Epstein. 1993. A causal model of health status and satisfaction with medical care. *Medical Care* 31 (1): 84–94.

Hunt, S. M., S. P. McKenna, and J. A. McKewen. 1980. A quantitative approach to perceived health status: A validation study. *Journal of Epidemiology and Community Health* 34: 281–85.

Kane, R. L. 1997. *Understanding Health Care Outcomes Research*. Gaithersburg, MD: Aspen Publishers.

Laitenen, J. 1976. Acupuncture and transcutaneous electric stimulation for the treatment of chronic sacrolumbalgia and ischialgia. *American Journal of Chinese Medicine* 4: 169.

MacDonald, A. J. R., K. D. Macrae, B. R. Master, et al. 1983. Superficial acupuncture in the relief of chronic low back pain. *Ann Coll Surg Engl* 65: 44.

Mishima, M., Y. Oku, S. Muro, T. Hirai, K. Chin, M. Ohi, M. Makagawa, M. Fujita, K. Sato, K. Shimada, S. Yamaoka, Y. Oda, N. Asai, H. Sagawa, and K. Kuno. 1996. Relationship between dyspnea in daily life and psycho-physiologic state in patients with chronic obstructive pulmonary disease during long-term domiciliary oxygen therapy. *Internal Medicine* 35 (6): 453–58.

Parkerson, G. F. J., W. E. Broadhead, and C. K. Tse. 1990. The Duke health profile: A 17-item measure of health and dysfunction. *Medical Care* 28: 1056.

Patrick, D. L., and R. A. Deyo. 1989. Generic and disease-specific measures in assessing health status and quality of life. *Medical Care* 27 (3): S217–32.

Patton, M, Q. 1980. *Qualitative Evaluation Methods*. Beverly Hills, CA: Sage.

Price, D. D., P. A. McGrath, R. Rafii, and B. Buckingham. 1983. The validation of visual analogue scales as ratio scale measures for chronic and experimental pain. *Pain* 17: 45–56.

Price, D. D., and S. W. Harkins. 1987. The combined use of visual analogue scales and experimental pain in providing standardized assessment of clinical pain. *Clin J Pain* 3: 3–11.

Rousseau, D. 1985. Issue of level in organizational research: Multilevel and cross level perspectives. *Research in Organizational Behavior* 7: 1–37.

Ware, J., and R. D. Hayes. 1988. Methods for measuring patient satisfaction with specific medical encounters. *Medical Care* 26: 393.

Ware, J. E., Jr., and C. D. Sherbourne. 1992. The MOS 36-item short-form health survey (SF-36): Conceptual framework and item selection. *Medical Care* 30 (6): 473–83.

6

Business Aspects of Integrative Health Care Programs

The survival of an integrative health care program requires that attention be paid to the business aspects of the program as it is developed and implemented. Because integrative programs are based on a new paradigm of care, leadership commitment to the program is essential. This chapter discusses this commitment, as well as concerns that arise when deciding on program structure, budgeting for the program, and marketing. Also described is the development of an alternative pharmacy offering herbal preparations, homeopathic remedies, and nutritional supplements—one of the largest single business concerns for an integrative program.

Leadership Commitment

As noted in earlier chapters, the commitment of both administrative and clinical leaders to the integration of alternative and complementary therapies is crucial to the program's success. Leaders need to believe in the philosophical premise that people have the right to the entire array of reputable health care options available to them; that is, the best of conventional care integrated with the best of alternative and complementary healing therapies. This commitment is especially important because leaders throughout the organization influence the various business aspects of the program, such as resource allocation, staffing, and insurer relations. For example, with the commitment of administration, recruitment of competent providers of care becomes possible.

Resistance within the organization or community may necessitate setting up the integrative program as a separate entity, at least in the initial stages. A separate, committed leadership structure will keep the established power groups within the organization from demanding that the program be stopped before it has a chance to succeed. If the program has an influential board, the members can help to deflect criticism of the program during its development. Administrative and clinical leaders need to give unequivocal support; they cannot give verbal support in meetings about the program and then remain silent when the program is discussed in general meetings. Furthermore, in order for the integration of alternative and complementary therapies to be viewed as receiving total support from the organization and to fund program continuation and expansion, the integrative program's external fundraising must be coordinated and implemented from a central source.

Program Structure

As with any health care program, a business structure underlies the integrative care program. Factors in determining the best initial structure for the program are the organization's political climate, the physical environment in which the program is carried out, and the practitioners who deliver care. The way an organization addresses each of these elements can greatly influence the success of the program.

The Political Climate

As has been mentioned throughout this book, many members of the conventional health care community are skeptical about the need for alternative and complementary therapies, as well as the benefits of integrating these therapies into allopathic models. The first consideration in developing a structure is whether the business factors (finances, marketing, and so on) of the project need to be insulated from outside influences that could inhibit its growth. For example, it works well for many programs, at least in the initial stages, to be separate from the existing structure of the hospital or group practice network.

Physical Environment

A second important consideration for developing a business structure is where the integrative health care program will be instituted first. It can begin with one demonstration site, multiple sites of similar size, or one large central site with smaller satellite sites in various service areas. That decision will depend on the system's mission, the program's mission, and budget limitations. For example, if the overall organization has a mission to provide services to the poor or underserved, then there needs to be a satellite site in an area that serves that population. If sites are limited to more affluent areas, the program is out of sync with its mission and becomes more difficult to defend.

It is probably best to begin with one small site because there are always refinements that need to be made with any new program and a smaller site can serve as a demonstration model. Practitioners and people in the community can observe integrative care and gradually become more comfortable with it. The initial site need not be a separate one; the program can begin with incorporation of alternative and complementary therapies into an existing program.

Site Ownership

Once the number of sites has been established, it is important to decide who the owner(s) of each will be. Multiple sites can be wholly owned by the overall organization or group practice network, or they can be owned jointly with others. The obvious advantage of total ownership is direct quality control. The potential advantage of joint ownership with program participants (for example, physicians) is that they have an incentive to be more productive and are more likely to have a team-player philosophy of interaction. This is an important consideration because the initial cadre of practitioners for the program will be obtained through a highly competitive process. Experts in integrative health care are rare at this point, and they are being sought actively by many organizations. Allowing independent and competent practitioners an active role in participating in the business, and reaping the rewards or suffering the setbacks, can make joining a specific program more appealing. The hybrid model in which the employee is a partner and, therefore, exposed to upside profits and downside risks can be attractive to the organization as well. The full employment model, in which practitioners are employees who assume no risk related to financial outcomes or productivity, is risky in program development.

Practitioners

An integrative health care program will ultimately only be as good as those providing care. Therefore, it is necessary to attract qualified practitioners who already practice alternative therapies or integrative care and encourage practitioners within the organization to become knowledgeable about alternative and complementary therapies (or to use those in which they may already be proficient).

Attracting Qualified Practitioners

Programs can begin with providers in the community who are already engaged in or are interested in providing integrative health care. The benefits an organized program can offer such providers include technical support; formation of a purchasing group for items such as herbs, homeopathic remedies, books, and acupuncture supplies; and billing services for their unique needs. Program administrators also can set up contracts with insurance carriers on behalf of provider participants. Developing such a network arrangement depends on the organization's economic goals, corporate philosophy regarding alternative providers, and regional politics. If an existing organization or system can incorporate nonconventional practitioners and permit them to participate in the referral process, integrating alternative providers into a network can be a viable option. Negotiations need to proceed with caution because many alternative providers have inadequate documentation and computer skills. Once these practitioners become part of a network, they will also need to understand contracts and participate in prospective and concurrent review. Many alternative providers have not had experience in these areas because their clients pay out-of-pocket for services.

Training In-house Practitioners in Integration

As mentioned in chapters 3 and 4, educating all employees about integrative care is one of the best ways to achieve buy-in and encourage a shift in attitude. Many organizations are surprised to find that many of their current practitioners and employees are competent, and often expert, in some of the alternative and complementary therapies. They can serve as valuable resources and educators. Others may be interested in learning some of the therapies and would do so with a small amount of encouragement from the organization.

Details That Make the Difference

The strategies a program uses to support decisions regarding the political climate, the physical distribution of the program, and the practitioners who deliver care can have an enormous impact on how the program as a whole is received. The following list provides suggestions for tying all elements of the program together with practice to make a unified whole:

- Telephone on-hold music should be consistent with the tone of an integrative health care program. Messages are not about the latest laser eye surgery available at the hospital, for example, but about helpful health tips and the integrative health care program and providers.
- The reading material or audiotapes and videotapes in the waiting room need to focus on educating patients about alternative therapies and ways in which they can become healthier. Newspapers are generally avoided because of their stressful content.
- Purified water and caffeine-free teas need to be available to patients and providers. It can be disconcerting to patients to

be in an environment that focuses on health and then see a provider with a soda containing highly-refined sugar and caffeine. Providers need to be aware about what patients may see them eating.

■ Individual audio facilities will allow patients to listen to music of their choice while waiting for their provider or for use during treatment.

■ The office should not smell like a medical clinic and the bathrooms need to be well ventilated.

■ Instead of the usual clinical gowns, people might be given cloth robes or kimonos and booties before seeing the provider, and there need to be mirrors in each room so patients may change to their street clothes comfortably after treatment.

■ While meeting code requirements, bathrooms should not look or feel clinical. Wallpaper and pictures on the walls need to promote a healing, restful atmosphere.

■ Floors need to be carpeted for sound control and kept clean. The patient care areas need to be as quiet as possible.

■ Staff need to make patients feel as if they are about to spend time at a marvelous spa-like facility.

■ Support staff need to wear uniforms in soft, muted colors.

■ Exam tables need to be wide, with comfortable cushions and elegant, inviting colors.

Budgetary Concerns

Developing a budget for integrative health care is not very different from developing one for conventional care. The most successful budget planning seems to be that which is divided into project phases: planning (including exploration costs); implementation (including marketing costs); and evaluation (including costs related to publicizing the project and its outcomes). The usual areas and items that need to be considered in developing a budget are provided in figure 6-1.

All integrative health care projects need to consider these budget areas, but actual costs will vary. Variations in cost depend on many factors, including the scope of the program, extent of existing structure, regional differences in provider compensation, and the resources within the organization.

FIGURE 6-1. Items to Consider in Developing a Budget

Planning

- Exploring other integrative health care projects, including relevant site visits for key project staff
- Books, articles, and tapes on integrative health care topics
- Salaries and other meeting costs for planning group
- Planning group attendance at selected integrative health care conferences
- Consultant costs for project planning and vision development
- Recruitment of alternative/complementary providers and/or network development
- Education and training of conventional providers regarding alternative therapies
- Facility construction and design or redesign improvements (aesthetic and regulatory agency needs), if required
- Rent or purchase costs for facility, if required
- Subscriptions to alternative health care journals
- Development of policies, procedures, and protocols
- Provider credentialing
- Insurance plan reimbursement needs
- Development of referral processes, case management processes, and utilization management plans

Implementation

- Baseline supplies for herbal, nutritional, and/or homeopathic products
- Insurance and malpractice concerns
- Equipment for alternative therapies (acupuncture needles, massage oils, and so on) and conventional care
- Salaries and fringe benefits for providers and office staff
- Usual office functions (supplies, phone, fax, billing, appointment scheduling)
- Allocated accreditation costs
- Marketing (local, regional, and national), as relevant
- Baseline and ongoing monitoring of project implementation and outcomes
- Continuous monitoring of compliance with regulatory requirements (local and national)
- Incentives to providers (patient load, product sales)
- High-quality answering service to maintain center focus
- Consultants for implementation phase

Evaluation

- Collection of outcomes data
- Analysis of implementation and outcomes data
- Reporting of data analysis (both facility-specific and general) at conferences and in journals
- Purchase of copyrighted data collection measures
- Consultants for evaluation phase (data analysis and reporting of results)

Mistakes to Avoid

Most often organizations do not budget sufficient funds for starting an integrative program; although the budget categories are not different, allocation of monies may be. In the initial phase, much financial support is needed for education and ongoing training of practitioners in selected therapies. These are not skills that most practitioners learn in their formal educational programs. In order for the practice of these therapies to be accepted, training should be obtained from respected programs and sources. Many of these programs have a short initial training period but require long-term continuing education, often supervised by an expert practitioner. A related expense is seeking out and buying literature and texts in alternative therapies and integrative care for the library, key practitioners, and administrative staff.

Administrators also need to understand that, if the integrative program is a group practice, higher ratios of both providers and support staff are needed in this type of program. Costs for high-tech equipment and procedures will be much lower, but since integrative practitioners may spend more time with people—to teach imagery or discuss care options—then the provider-patient ratio is often lower. Other costs that are often not thought of in the budget process are those for recruitment (expert integrative practitioners are uncommon) and physical improvements to the practice site. Training costs to prepare support staff for their new role are frequently forgotten as well.

Reimbursement Factors

One of the most important financial concerns for an integrative care program is the generation of a system of billing codes for alternative and complementary therapies. Without a system that specifically lists these therapies, practitioners tend to code an assessment or treatment into a category of conventional care that comes the closest to the alternative therapy. This practice may be construed as a way to receive compensation from an insurer that might otherwise refuse to pay for such services. Whether done from good intentions or simply from a lack of understanding, the use of creative coding in order to secure insurance reimbursement for a noncovered benefit is fraudulent. The legal aspects of this topic are discussed further in chapter 7.

In order to bridge the gap between alternative and conventional care, some groups have developed systems of alternative health care billing codes that are specific to the actual alternative procedures, use procedure descriptions, and define terms not usually used in conventional care. One of the most widely used set of billing codes is that generated by Alternative Link, based in New Mexico, which is being piloted at various sites in health plans throughout the country.

Alternative Link began by using the existing common procedure terminology (CPT) codes used by such professions as chiropractic, massage therapy, acupuncture, naturopathy, holistic medicine, and midwifery. These groups were selected because they had national certification standards, state licensing, and the ability to obtain malpractice insurance. Information from providers from several states was organized into categories. The result is a standardized computer-based system that identifies descriptors of service and terminology specific to alternative care. It is designed to fit into current medical information management systems. The CPT codes and the relative value units attached to them are being beta-tested by large populations of providers and several health insurance plans. Such a system will allow not only for the tracking of and payment for alternative health care, but also will permit analysis of cost and patient outcomes from conventional, alternative, and integrative care protocols.

Marketing Plan Development

A plan needs to be developed for marketing integrative health care to potential patients, health care professionals, community leaders, insurers, and the public at large. A marketing plan is the development of strategies to inform those who need or want integrative health care about the services included in the organization's program. The marketing plan includes information about integrative care, the specific alternative and complementary therapies that are available through the organization, and whether sales of homeopathic remedies, herbal preparations, and nutritional supplements are available to the general public.

A marketing plan is important because many people in the community may be actively seeking this type of care and even willing to pay for alternative care that is not covered by their insurance plans, yet are unaware of available services. It may sound odd to think that an organization will commit to integrating care yet be reluctant to market its program, but some who fear community skepticism or in-house divisiveness prefer to begin an integrative program without any publicity. Unfortunately, lack of effective marketing for any new program, regardless of the quality, contributes to program failure. An organization or group practice that chooses to initiate a program with little fanfare indicates a lack of commitment to the philosophy. In general, the public is supportive of credible organizations and practitioners providing integrative care, but marketing surveys and focus groups at a community level can be helpful. Marketing a program in integrative health care also can lead to positive outcomes for the organization as a whole, because in most cases integration of alternative therapies will be seen as a cutting-edge program sponsored by a progressive organization.

Some general marketing strategies for integrative care include the following:

- Use local radio and television to publicize the program and its providers.
- Design a unique logo that is consistent with the corporate logo design, but that indicates how the integrative health care program differs from conventional care.
- Design separate stationery for the program that incorporates the logo and is made from recycled paper.
- Have frequent meetings and discussions with community leaders to seek their participation.
- Develop affiliations with university-based health professional schools to encourage program credibility and gain access to other resources, such as data analysis assistance.
- Form an advisory board of influential community members and experts in alternative and complementary therapies.

Because of the nature of many alternative therapies, this board needs to include people from a broad range of demographic groups.

Development of an Alternative Pharmacy

One of the initial decisions that needs to be made if an integrative group project includes sales of herbal products, homeopathic remedies, and nutritional supplements is whether to develop an alternative pharmacy as part of its program. Because of the variation in production standards, review of such products is consistent with the provision of high-quality care. The organization or group practice can investigate products from several companies and decide on those that best meet its chosen criteria for quality. This is helpful to the public because the quality, dosing, stability, and expiration dates of herbal, homeopathic, and nutritional products can vary in the retail marketplace.

Because the development of an alternative pharmacy involves special business considerations that are separate from those of other parts of the program, this section describes each of these considerations in detail.

Regulation of Herbal Products

Herbal products are considered nutritional supplements by the Food and Drug Administration (FDA) and as such do not have as stringent production and claims standards as conventional pharmaceuticals. However, on April 24, 1998, the FDA proposed rules to make labeling for dietary supplements more informative, reliable, and uniform. Currently, labeling is mandated by the Dietary Supplement Health and Education Act of 1994 (DSHEA). Under DSHEA, claims can be made regarding the effect on structure or functioning of the body, but not claims on treating, diagnosing, curing, or preventing disease. The proposal under review defines the criteria for structure/function claims, as well as the disease claims that currently are prohibited (U.S. Department of Health and Human Services 1998). At the time of this writing, these rules are expected to go into effect in 1999.

When the FDA attempted to tighten regulation of these products, many consumers and lobbyists representing the herbal industry opposed the action, arguing that these products should have a more liberal set of controls and limited restrictions so consumers could exercise their right to choose their own health products. The challenge is to determine a way in which the freedom of health care consumers can be respected, while protecting them against unsubstantiated health claims made by those selling and manufacturing herbal products.

Standards for Herbal Products

Standards for herbal products are uneven. For example, there are no standards for what vehicles (gel capsule, freeze-dried capsule, tablet, or tincture) should be used for any given herb. Also, there are no clear conventions for the best way of testing for the active ingredient considered to be key for clinical efficacy. Because of this lack of standardization, consumers have no way of knowing the concentration of the active ingredient, if any, that is actually present in each pill or teaspoon and in each lot of the product. While there are now labeling guidelines with regard to herbal products and the claims that they can make for efficacy, 200 mg of an herbal product from one manufacturer may not be equivalent to 200 mg of the same product made by another company. Further, an herbal preparation could be contaminated with microbials or tainted with other products that have medicinal properties.

Inclusion of Homeopathic Products

Production and licensing of homeopathic remedies is regulated by the FDA, so the concerns regarding herbal products do not apply to these remedies. The labeling can create some confusion, however. The clinical indications and dosage for each remedy are often on the label, but practitioners may recommend the products for uses and dosages other than those shown on the package. (This can be a source of confusion for a patient with an ear infection who is using a product labeled for use in teething.) Once again, the pharmacy committee needs to be educated about these products, which are not included in most conventional pharmacy programs.

Creating the Formulary

The practitioners who will be integrating the use of herbal, homeopathic, and nutritional products into care will need to develop an alternative formulary. This group needs to include the director of the pharmacy at the organization or, if a group practice, a pharmacist who is knowledgeable in the use of alternative products.

The group determines what alternative products will be used most commonly and reviews suppliers' materials for quality control. Although the group may choose to use products from different companies, each company selected needs to have random audit of its products and independent laboratory testing. Although the number of untoward reactions from alternative products is small, this collaboration between the practitioners and the pharmacist, in combination with oversight of quality control processes used by suppliers, ensures the reputable use of alternative products integrated into conventional care.

Collaboration with Other Pharmacists

It is quite important to assess the support of the organization's pharmacy staff and pharmacy committee. This may require educating the pharmacists about unfamiliar alternative products. If there is a great deal of resistance, administration needs to consider whether the part of the organization that integrates the use of alternative products needs to be separated initially from the mainstream services. Even if integration of alternative products is possible, the sale of those products may need to be a separate product line. It is important to remember that the formulary committee will need to approve the alternative formulary if it is to be used within the inpatient facility or other sites in the system.

Including Natural Pharmacists

There is a growing number of pharmacists and clinical pharma-
cologists interested in botanical and homeopathic medicine in
response to interest and demand for information from consumers. The Society for Natural Pharmacy in New York has
become the premier organization and clearinghouse for this
rapidly expanding group. Natural pharmacists are beginning to
be integrated into conventional pharmacies, especially in pharmacy chains. Physicians and other providers in the integrative
program will require the collaboration of these specialists to
check drug-botanical interactions, suggest combinations that
might best achieve the goals of a practitioner not trained in this
area, and answer questions about these products from patients
and professionals.

Natural pharmacists also are key to developing and maintaining formularies for health systems and insurers. At present,
formularies are developed in an often arbitrary fashion by professionals who lack the specific training to judge product quality, indications, and contraindications. Managed care companies
that are either developing formularies or catalogues available to
their insureds could fall prey to a decision-making process
based primarily on cost. Natural pharmacists can play an important role in helping large institutions avoid the potential dangers inherent in developing an institutional formulary.

Software and educational programs designed to supplement information from natural pharmacists and assist institutions with use of natural medicines are being developed. (For
examples, see appendix A.)

Storage and Sales of Products

Herbal, nutritional, and homeopathic products need to be stored
in a temperature-controlled environment to avoid degrading the
potency of the active ingredients. Also, many companies do not
place expiration dates on their products, so procedures need to
be in place for review of the currency of products. (This should
be brought to the attention of the public as well, because many
consumers buy products at other facilities over which the organization has no control.) The storage area for these products

should be segregated, with only one egress and ingress so that there is adequate inventory control. The number and qualifications of staff handling these products must be restricted. A software or manual system for recording and tracking sales should be accurate and easy to use; a system that provides inventory control and can be programmed for use in product ordering is essential.

Education of Staff and Practitioners

Patients will have many questions regarding these products and their uses, even if practitioners think they have already reviewed all of the essential information during consultation. Other staff, including those in checkout, discharge, or sales, need to be adequately trained to respond appropriately to patient questions. More often than not, patients will purchase products other than those recommended by their provider because nutritional supplements and homeopathic remedies do not require prescriptions. It is important that written information is available for patients and staff and that staff are taught to refrain from making suggestions that border on prescribing without a license. In addition to having the usual sales capabilities, it can be a valuable service to have a phone-order capability for people who wish to continue use of a product, but do not need a provider visit. In general, one of the most important points to address with staff is that while it is tempting to encourage good salesmanship in order to increase revenues, the mission of integrative health care is to encourage responsible self-empowerment. Staff and practitioners need reminders that they are part of a health care team and not a retail sales force.

While organizational policy may be to discount products or dispense products without cost to those who cannot afford them, a clear collection policy for those who do pay is key. In this sense, staff should treat the matter as a retail sale and not be allowed to decide independently to extend credit or accept partial payment. Practitioners may not be accustomed to the retail environment and may find their role in this regard awkward; however, sales of products for which full cost is not received can amount to quite a bit in lost revenue or can add substantially to the work of accounts receivable if not adequately controlled.

Sales of alternative products offer a new way of expanding income generation for both institutions and providers. Recently, there has been a shift to give incentives to providers based on various factors, including productivity and income generated for the facility or group practice. However, retail products present a difficult situation for practitioners because their sales represent a potential for conflict of interest. One way to address this is to remove product sales from an individual practitioner's incentive pool and place the revenues in a general account that benefits the entire group or organization or that is not included in incentive calculations. Another possibility is to carefully monitor product sales by provider and examine those of any provider who appears to be a high user of these products. Also, a decision needs to be made concerning the most appropriate way to allocate the income derived from refill or independent sales; that is, those that result from patients or consumers initiating the order with or without practitioner recommendation.

Sales of Additional Related Products

Many organizations that provide integrative services find they can provide a very valuable service and generate additional revenue by offering for sale books or tapes on topics helpful to patients, such as nutrition for diabetics or relaxation tapes. This is because people are often highly motivated to make changes that might benefit their health while they are there in the practitioner's office. Patients view the availability of these materials as a service because they know that these resources have been screened by the program. Many items can be obtained from the suppliers at a discount; selling the materials at full price allows the program to recoup costs involved and generate a small profit.

Conclusion

The business aspects of an integrative health care program, including leadership, program structure, budgeting, marketing, and legal requirements (which are examined in the next chapter), are as important to success as the delivery of care, although these aspects are sometimes overlooked or poorly planned. An alternative pharmacy may pose the greatest number of challenges as a separate entity within the program.

Reference Cited

U.S. Department of Health and Human Services. 1998. FDA proposes rules to make claims for dietary supplements more informative, reliable and uniform. Press release, April 24. On-line: http://www.fda.gov.

7

Legal and Regulatory Issues in Integrative Health Care

Janet Kornblatt, JD, MPH, MA

The practice of integrative health care is characterized by the same administrative, regulatory, legal, and ethical considerations as any conventional health care practice. There is, however, one fundamental difference: the detractors of alternative and complementary therapies are themselves members of the health care establishment. Therefore, practitioners of alternative and complementary therapies may face seemingly authoritative claims that the treatments they offer are ineffective, if not harmful. They may be confronted with assertions that treatment standards are lacking; that they are charlatans (or worse) unleashed on an unsuspecting public.

The most effective way to counter such allegations is to ensure that the practice of alternative and complementary therapies:

- Complies with all federal, state, and local licensure and regulatory schemes
- Articulates and adheres to clearly documented quality assurance mechanisms
- Continually refines its provider-patient relationships
- Has defined, clear risk management policies and procedures of which all staff members are aware and to which they conform at all times

■ Develops close working relationships with insurers and managed care organizations
■ Implements a comprehensive and effective marketing and public relations strategy

There is no one blueprint to avoid legal pitfalls and respond to legal problems once they arise. This chapter, which applies to both institution-based and group practice situations, presents a broad overview of the key regulatory and legal issues involved in developing an integrative health care practice.

Regulatory Concerns

As an increasing number of Americans turn to alternative therapies for the treatment of health care problems, the providers of these therapies will find themselves under intense scrutiny. Therefore, they must take all necessary measures to conform to any existing professional standards and be able to document such compliance. Although these requirements are no more onerous than those imposed on conventional health care practitioners, adherence is potentially more important in the area of integrative health care because the regulations are enforced by those who may not have a clear understanding of alternative and complementary therapies.

Facility Issues

The first task is to identify all local codes, such as building codes, and state laws for health facilities, which must be satisfied whether the organization owns, leases, or renovates its facility. Points to consider are:

■ Handicapped access
■ Requirements of the Occupational Safety and Health Administration (OSHA)
■ Disposal of hazardous waste
■ Radiation shielding
■ Fire laws

- Ingress and egress for patients and staff
- Requirements for laboratory areas
- Adequacy of parking
- Condition of elevators
- Sufficient space for files and record retention areas
- Provision of or access to rooms for audiovisual equipment and staff training

Also important are the provision of natural light, sound proofing, comfortable waiting spaces, and adequate restrooms.

All required building permits must be obtained, as must any variances or permission for any alterations to the physical plant. Also, organizations that are accredited by the Joint Commission on Accreditation of Healthcare Organizations need to notify that group of renovations to the physical structure.

Licensing, Credentialing, and Scope of Practice Concerns

The need to identify and comply with all federal, state, and local licensure requirements applies to staff members as well as the physical plant. The biggest problem for practitioners of alternative and complementary therapies appears to be challenges to their credentials and licensure.

Usually, it is wise for the organization to advise the local medical licensing board, preferably in writing, of its intention to integrate alternative and complementary therapies into its practice. It may even be prudent to request a written acknowledgment (amounting to approval) of this information. Boards may decline to provide such a response, claiming that they do not provide "advisory opinions," meaning in the absence of any existing problem or conflict they are not going to offer any judgments. Even without a response, keeping the board advised of changes and developments in organizational practice may prove helpful in the event of any subsequent allegations of substandard care by local physicians or patients.

Keeping an open line of communication with the local board is always sound policy. Maintaining regular (even if infrequent) contact with the licensing board before problems arise lets the board know that an organization is practicing responsibly and with respect for the board's jurisdiction and judgment. It also is usually advisable to maintain a low profile. If certain providers in the organization's community have questionable practices, crusading on their behalf or aligning the organization with them may be political suicide. Battles should be chosen carefully. All relevant boards (for example, naturopathic, homeopathic, osteopathic, or dental) should be identified and contacted. Organizations also need to be sensitive to any turf battles that may exist between the various boards and to exercise discretion when dealing with them.

A frequent problem for health care practitioners is being called before a state board simply for practicing alternative and complementary therapies in medicine, nursing, or another discipline. Scope of practice statutes that exist in an organization's geographic area should be determined. Some states have laws protecting physicians from being investigated by state medical boards for practicing alternative and complementary medicine. The organization needs to ascertain what is permitted by state law and applicable boards, as well as the general climate in that state toward practitioners of the various healing therapies. There may be no formal standards in certain areas of practice, but there may be individuals with recognized expertise and reputation who can legitimize such practice by others. Obtaining the approval of such individuals for either a particular program, a particular practitioner, or both is always advisable. By doing so, the organization has identified a "gold standard" to which it can demonstrate that it has conformed should its practice be challenged.

Different issues may arise with different types of practices. Practitioners of acupuncture, osteopathic manipulation, and homeopathy are the easiest to credential, because there are existing "standards" and individuals capable of conducting some type of peer review. However, there also may be competing boards for the same area of practice. For example, various standards of care exist for acupuncture; one set is promulgated by the National Commission for the Certification of Acupuncturists, another by the American Association of Acupuncture and Oriental Medicine, and yet another by the American Academy of Medical Acupuncture. Standards for alternative pharmacologic therapies and drug substitutes such as herbal preparations, vitamins, and minerals vary. The organization should identify all reputable accredited organizations or individuals in a given practice area and keep in close contact with them on a continuing basis. In the event that difficult situations arise, an ongoing and current relationship may make these organizations and/or individuals more willing to speak on the organization's behalf.

Whenever possible and desirable, clinical privileges in a hospital setting should be obtained for alternative practitioners. Organizations need to be particularly careful in credentialing individuals who will practice alternative or complementary therapies under their auspices. All licenses, certification, and references need to be scrutinized and verified. Furthermore, providers who will practice in areas that are not formally licensed or certified (for example, yoga or tai chi masters) need to be directly and closely supervised by a licensed health care professional. All alternative practitioners should be particularly careful not to exceed the scope of their specific area of practice.

Federal Standards

In addition to the local and state regulatory concerns already discussed, the integrative health care project must adhere to all applicable federal laws and regulations. Federal agencies oversee controls in medications and medical devices, hazardous materials and wastes, reimbursement, and conflicts of interest.

Use of Medications and Devices

The Food and Drug Administration (FDA) strictly regulates drugs and medical devices (such as acupuncture needles and prostheses). The rules for physician prescribing are fairly clear, but the ability of nonphysician providers to write prescriptions can vary. In regard to herbs, vitamins, and nutritional supplements, the FDA has determined that such products qualify as foods and not drugs. However, on April 24, 1998, the FDA proposed rules to make claims for dietary supplements more informative, reliable, and uniform. Currently, labeling is mandated by the Dietary Supplement Health and Education Act of 1994 (DSHEA). Under DSHEA, claims can be made regarding a supplement's effect on structure or functioning of the body, but claims on the treatment, diagnosis, cure, or prevention of disease are not allowed. The proposal under review defines the criteria for structure/function claims, as well as the disease claims that are currently prohibited (U.S. Department of Health and Human Services 1998). At the time of this writing, these rules are expected to go into effect in 1999. In the meantime, practitioners should determine whether they are "recommending" or "prescribing" such treatments and what they may or may not claim to be the benefits. It should always be determined whether such substances are found in any applicable managed care formulary.

Infection Control

Every organization must have arrangements for the disposal of hazardous wastes within its facility, for biological pickup to remove hazardous waste from the premises, and for maintaining an approved site at which such wastes are safely deposited. Contingency plans also must be in place, particularly with regard to exposures related to the provision of services. Responses to incidents such as a needle stick to an employee must be well rehearsed. There also should be a clear policy for the vaccination of employees against certain communicable diseases such as hepatitis B. All plans must be clear, simple, and posted prominently. In addition, it is prudent to have all employees read and sign copies of these plans and to note in each personnel file that this information was received, reviewed, and understood.

Medicare and Medicaid

All providers need to refer to Medicare and Medicaid for guidelines as to what constitutes acceptable practice modalities. Those treatments for which such reimbursement is available tend to be considered "legitimate." If a participating Medicare provider offers a treatment that is not covered by

Medicare, that provider must advise the patient that he or she will be receiving an uncovered service that must be paid out-of-pocket. In these cases, the organization should have a clearly worded form explaining that, according to Medicare regulations, Medicare pays for only those services it deems to be "reasonable and necessary" and that the organization believes Medicare will deny payment for any of several reasons (which may be identified on the form). This form needs to be signed by the patient and the signature witnessed. When filing Medicare claims, the services rendered should be clearly and accurately described. Descriptions should never be adjusted to ensure coverage—this is clearly a fraudulent practice.

Conflicts of Interest

The Stark Amendment prohibits referrals by any provider to a facility or ancillary service in which that provider has a financial interest. Compliance with the provisions of the Stark Amendment can be extremely difficult. It is important for organizations to seek counsel before merging with, investing in, or joining any referral network. Failure to comply with this amendment can have serious ramifications.

Pharmacy Issues

If an organization plans to establish an on-site herbal or homeopathic pharmacy or other dispensary, the planning group should check state and local pharmacy laws to determine whether the planned activities constitute operation of a pharmacy under applicable state and local regulations. No prescription or alternative medications (other than small samples) should be provided to patients without first verifying that it is acceptable to do so in a given area. Some states have laws providing that practitioners can dispense only to patients of the organization and that dispensing to others subjects them to all state pharmacy laws. Consideration should be given to the possibility that providing medications, homeopathic remedies, herbal preparations, and/or nutritional supplements may increase the chances of being named in any lawsuit based on an adverse reaction to the product provided.

Another consideration with over-the-counter products (drugs, vitamins, herbs, nutritional supplements) is the issue of practitioner control. Patients may obtain certain medications or remedies at the facility and any number of other medications or remedies outside its premises. If adverse reactions or interactions occur, there may be medical and legal ramifications. In addition, if there is an on-site pharmacy, patients may try to purchase substances they have read about or heard recommended by practitioners other than facility staff. Some type of control mechanisms, even for substances for which prescriptions are not technically required, needs to be implemented.

If a hospital develops an alternative medicine formulary, care should be taken to select only those herbs, vitamins, and minerals that have legitimate claims to efficacy and to ensure that such products are recommended appropriately. Research into manufacturing standards, quality, and consistency of each product should be conducted as with any pharmaceutical-grade product, and dispensing should follow the manufacturer's recommendations or those of another authoritative source that can be documented.

Practice Management

Practice management deals with the day-to-day activities that take place to ensure that the highest quality of care is delivered with the minimum of liability exposure. Organizations that are instituting integrative care projects need to be aware of the most important activities for maintaining practices that are legally sound. These activities include documentation, communication, informed consent, and supervision of practitioners.

Documentation

The necessity of maintaining accurate, up-to-date documentation of all phases of care for both medical and legal reasons is familiar to all health care practitioners. One must be able to retrace all steps taken in treatment, whether conventional or alternative, in case the efficacy or legality of a procedure is questioned. The importance of good documentation cannot be overemphasized, and any system for documentation needs to be consistent throughout the organization. Thus, consideration must be given to both format and content.

Format of Patient Records

The most important provider tool is the patient record. The formal, structured, documentation methodology used in conventional health care needs to be adapted for alternative and complementary therapies. The recommended model is the problem-oriented medical record (POMR). The best records are generally deemed to be those that follow the SOAP (Subjective, Objective, Assessment, Plan) format. For example, a patient record compiled by a physician or nurse practitioner may read as follows:

Subjective symptoms: Chief complaint—aching muscle pain, fatigue

Objective observations: Clear nasal drainage; HEENT (head, eyes, ears, nose, and throat), chest, abdomen, skin, nodes unremarkable; patient on no medications

Assessment: Viral syndrome

Plan: RX—standardized extract of echinacea, 1 clove garlic daily until symptoms subside. DX—None at present. Patient education—Follow up in 3 days or PRN for temperatures greater than 100.5° F. Possible allergic reaction to herb, need to call if still feeling bad in 3 to 5 days; discussed use of herbs vs. antibiotics. Garlic could irritate stomach.

Records must be clear and legible and should provide other practitioners with all the necessary information to ensure continuity of patient care. When providing alternative or complementary therapies, practitioners need to be clear about what is being done and why; for example, why a particular homeopathic remedy was chosen, which specific acupuncture points were used and why, and so on.

Checklists have proved very useful in adapting the POMR and SOAP methodologies, especially if a practitioner is overwhelmed and time is a problem. If a patient fills out a conventional intake or assessment form, the practitioner should read it. Often, patients will include information, such as over-the-counter medications or vitamin supplements, on a form that they will not verbally mention having taken. Also, a separate medication record, which may include herbs, vitamins, and homeopathic remedies as an integral part of the list, needs to be maintained in the patient record.

Follow-Up and Instructions

Basically, all conversations regarding risks, alternatives, instructions, and necessary follow-up should be documented. Practitioners need to review, and indicate that they have reviewed, all reports and test results pertaining to a patient. Preprinted instructions should be available for more common conditions and therapies; patients can then sign a document to acknowledge receipt and understanding of that information. Required telephone calls to determine patient condition after any outpatient procedures such as acupuncture should be documented in the patient's record. A tickler system should be in place to remind patients of the need for return visits or re-examination. Efforts to reach patients who fail to return for follow-up visits also should be included in the record.

Telephone Calls

In addition to documenting practitioner follow-up calls, the organization needs to have a procedure for documenting all pertinent patient inquiries. Offices should have some type of mechanism for either dictation by a practitioner of telephone contacts or recording them in writing. There must also be a means to cross-check requests for prescription refills with the patient's record.

Communication

The development of honest and open provider-patient partnerships is as important as good documentation. This is clearly the first line of defense against malpractice claims; it is generally unhappy patients who bring lawsuits. It is impossible to overemphasize the importance of keeping the lines of communication open, respecting a patient's intelligence, providing patients with all available information (whether positive or negative), and consulting with patients on all issues and decisions that affect their well-being. Something as simple as always returning patient phone calls may be the most important component of treatment and the most effective way to keep practitioners and organizations out of court.

The first step is to identify any concerns the patient has, whatever the cause. These may be regarding pain or psychosocial, financial, or other concerns and should be addressed as thoroughly as possible. If a patient has concerns about an alternative therapy suggested for treatment, an appropriate referral for a second opinion may be necessary. If the referral is declined, this needs to be documented in the patient record. When a patient elects to pursue alternative therapies in the absence of conventional therapies, or alternative therapies in combination with conventional therapies, the record must reflect this and a written patient consent must be obtained.

If the plan of care includes alternative and complementary therapies, the practitioner must explain the purpose or reason for their inclusion to the patient, define the responsibilities of both the patient and the provider, estimate the duration of treatment, and outline a financial arrangement. When necessary, it should be made clear to the patient that the therapy selected is unproven, that no adequate data exist to support its efficacy, and that some aspects of treatment may be considered "unconventional" by the conventional health care community. This is particularly significant when patients elect to forgo an accepted conventional therapy with a likelihood of cure in favor of an alternative therapy. Patients must be provided with all available information and advised to consult with all available resources. In some situations, an actual written physician-patient contract may be advisable.

Informed Consent

Informed consent is not merely one discussion, but rather a process that culminates in patients signing a form, in the presence of a witness (usually a staff member), that indicates acceptance of the care or services to be provided. Provision of all available information to patients, along with patient participation in the decision-making process, are the only valid methods by which a truly informed consent can be obtained. Patients should always be treated with respect.

All consent forms must be clear and use simple language. It may be best to provide individual forms for each treatment, particularly if the treatment is invasive. The consent form should be formatted as much like a contract as possible. It indicates that patients knowingly and willingly assume responsibility for and are active participants in treatment.

Supervision of Practitioners

Patient records should be reviewed and senior practitioners should be on the premises and available for consultation, particularly where this is required by local licensing laws. An overconfident or overeager practitioner of any therapy should never be allowed to overstep legal bounds or the practice limitations that have been imposed by the organization.

All staff members need to maintain their credentials as required, and all licenses must be kept current. Practitioners must be given the necessary time and financial support to attend ongoing training workshops and to maintain their licenses. Memberships in professional organizations are important and financial support for them should be available.

Protocols should exist for every type of practitioner within the organization and be checked constantly for compliance with changing requirements as well as to reflect any new developments in the field. These protocols must be written clearly and reviewed periodically by all providers at the facility. When appropriate, provider input into the development of protocols should be sought. However, the ultimate decisions are those of the project director and/or administration. Also, concurrent multidisciplinary review of current and specific cases is mandatory.

Coordination with Legal Counsel

Because the legal and regulatory requirements for integrative health care can become complex, it is important for the project director to maintain open communication with the organization's legal counsel. This may comprise in-house attorneys, those who are dedicated to the integrative health care arrangements, or those who handle threatened or ongoing malpractice lawsuits. Information and explanatory materials about the project should be reviewed by the proper counsel throughout the planning, implementation, and evaluation phases of the project. Not only can attorneys make suggestions about any plans that may be legally problematic, but also they can answer questions about regulatory and legal requirements so precautions can be taken beginning with the initial phase of the project. Keeping them apprised of the project's plans and progress also means they will be better prepared to deal with any complications that arise in future. The main areas in which legal counsel can provide the most help are:

- Litigation
- Termination of care
- Referrals and coordination of care
- Malpractice insurance
- Managed care relationships
- Employment issues

Litigation

In the event of a lawsuit, instructions should be obtained immediately from the appropriate counsel. Staff should be warned never to discuss threatened or actual litigation with anyone and never to proceed without benefit of counsel. The specific patient involved should never be discussed with either the patient's lawyer or opposing counsel without specific written permission from the patient. Nothing should be done, even something as seemingly innocuous as responding to subpoenas for medical records, without consulting an attorney first.

The organization's and/or practitioner's malpractice carrier should be notified immediately if it is not already aware of the situation, applicable records should be segregated, and all staff should be advised of the litigation. A separate file regarding the litigation should be kept that must not be integrated with the patient record under any circumstances. Never, under any circumstances, should an existing patient record be altered.

Termination of Patient Relationships

Should it become necessary to terminate a relationship with a patient, great care should be taken in doing so. Many patients who seek alternative therapies are those who have found that conventional health care can provide no relief or who believe they have been abandoned by the conventional medical community in one way or another.

If it becomes necessary to terminate a relationship, it is important to avoid claims of patient abandonment. The patient should be advised in clear, understandable terms that the organization can no longer provide services and a date for the termination of services should be identified. The practitioner or staff member should offer to transfer patient records and make appropriate referrals. A certified return-receipt notification outlining all of these points should be sent to the patient.

Referrals and Coordination of Care

Referrals must be made in writing and documented in the patient record as appropriate and as requested by the patient. This is particularly true when a patient is refusing a conventional form of therapy. Communication between referring practitioners and referral physicians is crucial, even in situations in which the patient will not be returning to the original practitioner. Physicians who are providing concurrent therapies should be included in the communication loop. Referrals for consultations and second opinions should be made when appropriate and documented. Coordination of care is particularly important for practitioners of integrative care because of the excessive scrutiny to which alternative or complementary therapies may be subjected.

Malpractice Insurance

Most insurance carriers appear to be supportive of integrative health care and offer appropriate coverage. If the organization has existing coverage for conventional care, the carrier should be advised in advance of the institution of the integrative health care project and the addition of alternative or complementary services. Even if the only change is supervision of a practitioner of an alternative modality, the carrier should be notified. Insurance companies do not like surprises and will appreciate being informed in advance. A written record of the change in coverage for the provision of alternative or complementary therapies should be obtained from the carrier.

Various practitioners, including nurse practitioners, nurse midwives, or acupuncturists, should have their own malpractice policies. The need for this depends on their licensure, scope of practice, and ability to perform independently.

Managed Care Relationships

Relationships with insurance companies and managed care organizations may be difficult to forge, yet desirable. Contracts with insurance companies should spell out exactly what the company and the provider expect in relation to the provision of integrative services. If individual agreements regarding care to be rendered to specific patients are entered into, these must be in writing before the treatment is provided. Attorneys should be consulted before any contracts are signed.

Companies with which the organization already has contracts should be informed of the integration of alternative and complementary therapies. They will determine whether any separate or specific coding is applicable for these therapies. To avoid questions and audits, alternative and complementary services should be billed separately, and codes assigned to conventional therapies should not be used if they do not specifically apply. Meetings involving the project director, administration, legal counsel, and a representative from the insurers with which the organization has relationships ensure that everyone is aware of the adoption of integrative care and the arrangements for reimbursement.

Employment Issues

Attorneys need to check all benefits and retirement plans for conformity to existing state and federal laws, specifically with regard to eligibility and availability to personnel. When practitioners are hired, their contracts should be reviewed by qualified legal personnel and verified that the agreement is voluntary. It also should be determined whether the practitioners have any existing contracts or commitments and confirmed that these do *not conflict in any way*. Practitioners' potential or active involvement in pending or threatened litigation should be explored and all intellectual property issues clarified prior to retaining employees in any capacity.

Conclusion

When implementing an integrative health care project, it is important to cover all the legal bases. The project will invariably be held to a higher standard of practice, and this overview discusses only the key issues an organization may confront. Integrative care is still new territory, and it is best to overemphasize rather than overlook legal and regulatory requirements (which can change at a rapid rate). Legal counsel is an excellent resource in planning for and meeting necessary requirements and in avoiding potential pitfalls.

Reference Cited

U.S. Department of Health and Human Services. 1998. FDA proposes rules to make claims for dietary supplements more informative, reliable and uniform. Press release, April 24. On-line: http://www.fda.gov.

APPENDIX A

Resources

This appendix provides readers with an array of resources with which to learn more about alternative and complementary therapies and the ways they can be integrated into conventional health care. An assortment of books, journal articles, Web sites, conferences, and organizations is provided to help readers begin the exploration into this exciting area.

No attempt has been made to make this list all-inclusive; rather, it furnishes a sampling of different areas, grouped in specific and general areas, as a starting point. The resources in each area are growing at an exponential rate, and readers are encouraged to develop their own libraries and networks of resources.

Books and Articles

General

Dossey, B. M. *American Holistic Nurses' Association Core Curriculum for Holistic Nursing.* Gaithersburg, MD: Aspen, 1997.

Dossey, B. M., L. Keegan, C. E. Guzzetta, and L. G. Kolkmeier. *Holistic Nursing: A Handbook for Practice.* 2d ed. Gaithersburg, MD: Aspen, 1995.

Dossey, L. How should alternative therapies be evaluated? *Alternative Therapies in Health and Medicine* 1 (2): 6–10, 79–85, 1995.

Eisenberg, D. M., et al. Unconventional medicine in the United States. *The New England Journal of Medicine* 328 (4): 246–51, 1993.

Gazella, K. A., ed. *Professional's Guide to Natural Healing.* Green Bay, WI: Impakt Communications, 1997.

Gordon, J. *Manifesto for a New Medicine: Your Guide to Healing Partnerships and the Wise Use of Alternative Therapies.* Reading, MA: Addison Wesley, 1996.

Lerner, M. *Choices in Healing: Integrating the Best of Conventional and Complementary Approaches to Cancer.* Cambridge, MA: MIT Press, 1994.

Spiegel, D. Effect of psychosocial treatment on survival of patients with metastatic breast cancer. *Lancet* 2: 888–91, October 14, 1989.

Standish, L. J., C. Calabrese, C. Reeves, N. Polissar, S. Bain, and T. O'Donnell. A scientific plan for the evaluation of alternative medicine in the treatment on HIV/AIDS. *Alternative Therapies in Health and Medicine* 3 (2): 58–67, 1997.

Time-Life Books. *The Medical Advisor: The Complete Guide to Alternative and Conventional Treatments.* New York: Time-Life Books, 1996.

Weil, A. *Natural Health, Natural Medicine.* Boston: Houghton Mifflin, 1995.

———. *Spontaneous Healing.* New York: Knopf, 1995.

Workshop on Alternative Medicine, Chantilly, VA. *Alternative Medicine: Expanding Medical Horizons.* A report to the National Institutes of Health on Alternative Medical Systems and Practices in the United States. Washington, DC: U.S. Government Printing Office, 1992.

Acupressure

Gach, M. R. *Acupressure's Potent Points: A Guide to Self-Care for Common Ailments*. New York: Bantam, 1990.

Jarney, C., and J. Tindall. *Acupressure for Common Ailments*. New York: Fireside, 1991.

Acupuncture

Camp, V. The place of acupuncture in medicine today. *British Journal of Rheumatology* 34 (5): 404–6, 1995.

Carneiro, N. M., and S. M. Li. Acupuncture technique. *The Lancet* 354: 1577, 1995.

Chen, C. H., P. Chou, H. Hu, and J. J. Tsuei. Further analysis of a pilot study for planning an extensive clinical trial in traditional medicine—an example of acupuncture treatment for stroke. *American Journal of Chinese Medicine* 22 (2): 127–36, 1994.

Elkayam, O., S. B. Itzhak, E. Avrahami, Y. Meidan, N. Doron, I. Eldar, I. Keidar, N. Liram, and M. Yaron. Multidisciplinary approach to chronic back pain: Prognostic elements of the outcome. *Clinical and Experimental Rheumatology* 14: 281–88, 1996.

Erickson, R. J. Acupuncture for chronic pain: A study of its efficacy, and an evaluation of its effect on utilization of medical services in a prepaid health plan. *Medical Acupuncture* 7 (1): 5–10, 1995.

Helms, J. An overview of medical acupuncture. *Alternative Therapies in Health and Medicine* 4 (3): 35–45, 1998.

Jackson, A. Acupuncture and migraine. *Nursing Times* 91 (13): 64, 1995.

Lewith, G. T. Migraine: The complementary approaches considered. *Complementary Therapies in Medicine* 4: 26–30, 1996.

McLellan, A. T., D. S. Grossman, J. D. Blaine, and H. W. Haverkos. Acupuncture treatment for drug abuse: A technical review. *Journal of Substance Abuse Treatment* 10 (6): 569–76, 1993.

Podolsky, D. Nod to an ancient art: The FDA has OK'd acupuncture needles—and they could help you. *US News and World Report:* 78–80, May 13, 1996.

Schulte, E. Acupuncture: Where East meets West. *RN* 59 (10): 55–57, 1996.

Zwolfer, W., W. Keznickl-Hillebrand, A. Spacek, M. Cartellieri, and G. Grubhofer. Beneficial effect of acupuncture on adult patients with bronchial asthma. *American Journal of Chinese Medicine* 21 (2): 113–17, 1993.

Aromatherapy

Buckle, J. *Clinical Aromatherapy in Nursing.* San Diego: Singular Publishing Group, Inc., 1997.

Flanagan, N. The clinical use of aromatherapy in Alzheimer's patients. *Alternative and Complementary Therapies:* 377–80, 1995.

Walsh, D. Using aromatherapy in the management of psoriasis. *Nursing Standard* 11: 53–56, 1996.

Worwood, V. A. *The Complete Book of Essential Oils and Aromatherapy.* San Rafael, CA: New World Library, 1991.

Ayurvedic Medicine

Morrison, J. H. *The Book of Ayurveda.* New York: Simon & Schuster, 1995.

Herbal Preparations

Braeckman, J. The extract of *Serenoa repens* in the treatment of BPH: A multicenter open study. *Current Therapeutic Research* 55 (7): 776–85, 1994.

Champlault G., J. C. Patel, and A. M. Bonnard. A double-blind trial of an extract of the plant *Serenoa repens* in BPH. *British Journal of Clinical Pharmacology* 18: 461–62, 1984.

Fugh-Berman, A. Clinical trials of herbs. *Primary Care* 24 (4): 889–903, 1997.

Linde, K., G. Ramirez, C. D. Mulrow, A. Pauls, W. Weidenhammer, and D. Melchart. St. John's wort for depression: An overview and meta-analysis of randomized clinical trials. *British Medical Journal* 313: 253–57, 1996.

Lipp, F. J. The efficacy, history, and politics of medicinal plants. *Alternative Therapies in Health and Medicine* 2 (4): 36–41, 1996.

Murray, M. *The Healing Power of Herbs.* 2d ed. Rocklin, CA: Prima Publishing, 1995.

Warshafsky, S., R. S. Kamer, and S. L. Sivak. Effect of garlic on total serum cholesterol. *Annals of Internal Medicine* 119: 599–605, 1993.

Werbach, M. R., and M. T. Murray. *Botanical Influences on Illness: A Sourcebook of Clinical Research.* Tarzana, CA: Third Line Press, 1994.

Youngkin, E. Q., and D. S. Israel. A review and critique of common herbal alternative therapies. *Nurse Practitioner* 21 (10): 39–62, 1996.

Homeopathy

Cummings, S., and D. Ullman. *Everybody's Guide to Homeopathic Medicines.* New York: Putnam, 1991.

Davidson, J., R. M. Morrison, J. Shore, R. T. Davidson, and G. Bedayn. Homeopathic treatment of depression and anxiety. *Alternative Therapies in Health and Medicine* 3 (1): 46–49, 1997.

de Lange de Klerk, E. S., J. Blommers, D. J. Kuik, P. D. Bezemer, and L. Feenstra. Effect of homoeopathic medicines on daily burden of symptoms in children with recurrent upper respiratory infections. *British Medical Journal* 309: 1329–32, 1994.

Horrigan, B. Research, homeopathy, and therapeutic consultation (interview with David Reilly). *Alternative Therapies in Health and Medicine* 1 (4): 65–73, 1995.

Jacobs, J., M. Jimenez, S. S. Gloyd, J. L. Gale, and D. Crothers. Treatment of acute childhood diarrhea with homeopathic medicine: A randomized clinical trial in Nicaragua. *Pediatrics* 93 (5): 719–25, 1994.

Kleijnen, J., P. Knipschild, and G. Riet. Clinical trials of homeopathy. *British Medical Journal* 302: 316–23, 1991.

Mossad, S. B., M. L. Macknin, S. V. Medendorp, and P. Mason. Zinc gluconate lozenges for treating the common cold: A randomized double-blind placebo controlled study. *Annals of Internal Medicine*, 125: 2, 81–88, 1996.

Reilly, D., M. A. Taylor, N. G. Beattie, J. H. Campbell, C. McSharry, T. C. Aitchison, R. Carter, and R. D. Stevenson. Is evidence for homeopathy reproducible? *The Lancet* 344: 1601–6, 1994.

Zell, I., et al. Treatment of acute sprains of the ankle. *Journal of Natural Medicine* 7 (1): 1–6, 1989.

Imagery

Achterberg, J., B. Dossey, and L. Kolkmeier. *Rituals of Healing: Using Imagery for Health and Wellness.* New York: Bantam, 1994.

Dossey, B. Using imagery to help your patient heal. *American Journal of Nursing* 95 (6): 40–47, 1995.

Goleman, D., and J. Gurin, eds. *Mind/Body Medicine: How to Use Your Mind for Better Health.* Yonkers, NY: Consumer Reports Books, 1993.

Maguire, B. L. The effects of imagery on attitudes and moods in multiple sclerosis patients. *Alternative Therapies in Health and Medicine* 2 (5): 75–79, 1996.

Manyande, A., S. Berg, D. Gettins, C. Stanford, D. Phil, S. Mazero, D. F. Marks, and P. Salmon. Preoperative rehearsal of active coping imagery influences subjective and hormonal responses to abdominal surgery. *Psychosomatic Medicine* 57: 177–82, 1995.

Mast, D. E. Effects of imagery. *Image: Journal of Nursing Scholarship* 18 (3): 118–20, 1986.

Moody, L. E., M. Fraser, and H. Yarandi. Effects of guided imagery in patients with chronic bronchitis and emphysema. *Clinical Nursing Research* 2 (4): 478–86, 1993.

Naparstek, B. *Staying Well with Guided Imagery.* New York: Warner Books, 1994.

Pederson, C. Effect of imagery on children's pain and anxiety during cardiac catheterization. *Journal of Pediatric Nursing* 10 (6): 365–74, 1995.

Rancour, P. Interactive guided imagery with oncology patients. *Journal of Holistic Nursing* 12 (2): 148–54, 1994.

Rossman, M. *Healing Yourself: A Step-by-Step Program for Better Health Through Imagery.* New York: Walker, 1987.

Shames, K. H. Harness the power of guided imagery. *RN* 58 (8): 49–50, 67, 1996.

Stevens, R. Imagery: A strategic intervention to empower clients. Part I—review of research literature. *Clinical Nurse Specialist* 7 (4): 170–74, 1993.

Stevens, R. L. Imagery: A strategic intervention to empower clients. Part II—a practical guide. *Clinical Nurse Specialist* 7 (5): 235–40, 1993.

Syrjala, K. L., G. W. Donaldson, M. W. Davis, M. E. Kippes, and J. E. Carr. Relaxation and imagery and cognitive-behavioral training reduce pain during cancer treatment: A controlled clinical trial. *Pain* 63: 189–98, 1995.

Troesch, L. M., C. B. Rodehaver, B. Delaney, and B. Yanes. The influence of guided imagery on chemotherapy-induced nausea and vomiting. *Oncology Nursing Forum* 20 (8): 1179–85, 1993.

Music Therapy

Augustin, P., and A. A. Hains. Effect of music on ambulatory surgery patients' preoperative anxiety. *AORN Journal* 63 (4): 750–56, 1996.

Bailey, L. M. Music therapy in pain management. *Journal of Pain and Symptom Management* 1 (1): 25–27, 1986.

Beck, S. L. The therapeutic use of music for cancer-related pain. *Oncology Nursing Forum* 18 (8): 1327–37, 1991.

Boldt, S. The effects of music therapy on motivation, psychological well-being, physical comfort, and exercise endurance of bone marrow transplant patients. *Journal of Music Therapy* 33 (3): 164–88, 1996.

Brown, C. J., A. C. N. Chen, and S. F. Dworkin. Music in the control of human pain. *Music Therapy* 8 (1): 47–60, 1989.

Frank, J. M. The effects of music therapy and guided visual imagery on chemotherapy induced nausea and vomiting. *Oncology Nursing Forum* 12 (5): 47–52, 1985.

Froehlich, M. A. R. A comparison of the effect of music therapy and medical play therapy on the verbalization behavior of pediatric patients. *Journal of Music Therapy* 21 (1): 2–15, 1984.

Kaempf, G., and M. E. Amodei. The effect of music on anxiety. *AORN Journal* 50 (1): 112–18, 1989.

Maslar, P. The effect of music on the reduction of pain: A review of the literature. *The Arts in Psychotherapy* 13: 215–19, 1986.

McKinney, C. H., F. C. Tims, A. M. Kumar, and M. Kumar. The effect of selected classical music and spontaneous imagery on plasma-endorphin. *Journal of Behavioral Medicine* 20 (1): 85–99, 1997.

Schroeder-Sheker, T. Music for the dying: A personal account of the new field of music thanatology—history, theories, and clinical narratives. *Advances, The Journal of Mind-Body Health* 9 (1): 36–48, 1993.

Zimmerman, L., B. Pozehl, K. Duncan, and R. Schmitz. Effects of music in patients who had chronic cancer pain. *Western Journal of Nursing Research* 11 (3): 293–309, 1989.

Nutrition

Badmaev, V., M. Majeed, and R. A. Passwater. Selenium: A quest for better understanding. *Alternative Therapies in Health and Medicine* 2 (4): 59–67, 1996.

Bland, J. S. Psychoneuro-nutritional medicine: An advancing paradigm. *Alternative Therapies in Health and Medicine* 1 (2): 22–27, 1995.

―――. Phytonutrition, phytotherapy, and phytopharmacology. *Alternative Therapies in Health and Medicine* 2 (6): 73–76, 1996.

Bland, J. S., E. Barrager, R. G. Reedy, and K. Bland. A medical food-supplemented detoxification program in the management of chronic health problems. *Alternative Therapies in Health and Medicine* 1 (5): 62–71, 1995.

Clark, L. C., G. F. Combs, B. W. Turnbull, E. H. Slate, D. K. Chalker, J. Chow, L. S. Davis, R. A. Glover, G. F. Graham, E. G. Gross, A. Krongard, J. L. Lesher, K. Park, B. B. Sanders, C. L. Smith, and J. R. Taylor. Nutritional Prevention of Cancer Study Group. Effects of selenium supplementation for cancer prevention in patients with carcinoma of the skin: A randomized controlled trial. *Journal of the American Medical Association* 276 (24): 1957–63, 1996.

Gaby, A. R. The role of coenzyme Q10 in clinical medicine. Part II. Cardiovascular disease, hypertension, diabetes mellitus, and infertility. *Alternative Medicine Review* 1 (3): 168–73, 1996.

Godfrey, J. C., N. J. Godfrey, and S. G. Novick. Zinc for the common cold: Review of all clinical trials since 1984. *Alternative Therapies in Health and Medicine* 2 (6): 63–72, 1996.

Gould, K. L., D. Ornish, L. Scherwitz, S. Brown, R. P. Edens, M. J. Hess, N. Mullani, F. Dobbs, W. T. Armstrong, T. Merritt, T. Ports, S. Sparier, and J. Billings. Changes in myocardial perfusion abnormalities by positron emission tomography after long-term, intense risk-factor modification. *Journal of the American Medical Association* 274 (11): 894–901, 1995.

Greenberg, S. M., and W. H. Frishman. Coenzyne Q10: A new drug for myocardial ischemia? *Medical Clinics of North America* 72 (1): 243–58, 1988.

———. Co-enzyme Q10: A new drug for cardiovascular disease. *Journal of Clinical Pharmacology* 30: 596–608, 1990.

Kamikawa, T., A. Kobayashi, and T. Yamashita. Effects of coenzyme Q10 on exercise tolerance in chronic stable angina pectoris. *American Journal of Cardiology* 56: 247–51, 1985.

Mossad, S. B., M. L. Macknin, S. V. Medendorp, and P. Mason. Zinc gluconate lozenges for treating the common cold. *Annals of Internal Medicine* 125 (2): 81–88, 1996.

Murray, M. *Encyclopedia of Nutritional Supplements.* Green Bay, WI: Impakt Communications, 1996.

Ornish, D. *Dr. Dean Ornish's Program for Reversing Heart Disease.* New York: Random House, 1990.

Ornish, D., S. E. Brown, L. W. Scherwitz, J. H. Billings, W. T. Armstrong, T. A. Ports, S. M. McLanahan, R. L. Kirkeeide, R. J. Brand, and K. L. Gould. Can lifestyle changes reverse coronary heart disease? *The Lancet* 336: 129–33, 1990.

Stevens, N. G., A. Parsons, P. M. Schofield, F. Kelly, K. Cheeseman, M. J. Mitchinson, and M. J. Brown. Randomized controlled trial of vitamin E in patients with coronary disease: Cambridge Heart Antioxidant Study (CHAOS). *The Lancet* 347: 781–86, 1996.

Warshafsky, S., R. S. Kamer, and S. L. Sivak. Effect of garlic on total serum cholesterol. *Annals of Internal Medicine* 119: 599–605, 1993.

Youngkin, E. Q., and D. S. Israel. A review and critique of common herbal alternative therapies. *Nurse Practitioner* 21 (10): 39–62, 1996.

Reflexology

Crane, B. *Reflexology: The Definitive Practitioner's Manual.* Rockport, MA: Element, 1997.

Frankel, B. The effect of reflexology on baroreceptor reflex sensitivity, blood pressure and sinus arrhythmia. *Complementary Therapies in Medicine* 5: 80–84, 1997.

Norman, L. *Feet First: A Guide to Foot Reflexology.* New York: Fireside, 1988.

Oleson, T., and W. Flocco. Randomized controlled study of premenstrual symptoms treated with ear, hand, and foot reflexology. *Obstetrics and Gynecology* 82 (6): 906–11, 1993.

Spirituality

Bauer, T., and C. R. Barron. Nursing interventions for spiritual care. *Journal of Holistic Nursing* 13 (3): 268–69, 1995.

Dossey, L. *Healing Words: The Power of Prayer and the Practice of Medicine.* San Francisco: Harper, 1993.

———. *Prayer Is Good Medicine.* San Francisco: Harper, 1996.

Levin, J. S. How prayer heals: A theoretical model. *Alternative Therapies in Health and Medicine* 2 (1): 66–73, 1996.

Lewis, P. J. A review of prayer within the role of the holistic nurse. *Journal of Holistic Nursing* 14 (4): 308–15, 1996.

Therapeutic Touch

Heidt, P. Effect of therapeutic touch on the anxiety level of hospitalized patients. *Nursing Research* 30 (1): 32–37, 1981.

Keller, E., and V. M. Bzdek. Effects of therapeutic touch on tension headache pain. *Nursing Research* 35 (2): 101–6, 1986.

Kramer, N. A. Comparison of therapeutic touch and casual touch in stress reduction on hospitalized children. *Pediatric Nursing* 16 (5): 483–85, 1990.

Krieger, D. *Accepting Your Power to Heal: The Personal Practice of Therapeutic Touch*. Santa Fe, NM: Bear, 1993.

Macrae, J. *Therapeutic Touch: A Practical Guide*. New York: Alfred A. Knopf, 1988.

Meehan, T. C. Therapeutic touch and postoperative pain: A Rogerian research study. *Nursing Science Quarterly* 6 (2): 69–77, 1993.

Olson, M., N. Sneed, M. LaVia, G. Virella, R. Bonadonna, and Y. Michel. Stress-induced immunosuppression and therapeutic touch. *Alternative Therapies in Health and Medicine* 3 (2): 68–74, 1997.

Peck, S. D. E. The effectiveness of therapeutic touch for decreasing pain in elders with degenerative arthritis. *Journal of Holistic Nursing* 15 (2): 176–98, 1997.

Quinn, J. F. Therapeutic touch as energy exchange: Replication and extension. *Nursing Science Quarterly* 2 (2): 74–78, 1989.

Therapeutic Touch: Healing Through Human Energy Fields (series of three videos and one video for family caregivers). Available from HaelanWorks, 303/449-5790.

Wirth, D. P. The effect of non-contact therapeutic touch on the healing rate of full thickness dermal wounds. *Subtle Energies* 1 (1): 1–20, 1992.

Wirth, D. P., M. J. Barrett, and W. S. Eidelman. Non-contact therapeutic touch and wound re-epithelialization: An extension of previous research. *Complementary Therapies in Medicine* 94 (2): 187–92, 1994.

Wirth, D. P., J. T. Richardson, W. S. Eidelman, and A. C. O'Malley. Full thickness dermal wounds treated with non-contact therapeutic touch: A replication and extension. *Complementary Therapies in Medicine* 1 (3): 127–32, 1993.

Wirth, D. P., J. T. Richardson, R. D. Martinez, W. S. Eidelman, and M. E. Lopez. Non-contact therapeutic touch intervention and full-thickness cutaneous wounds: A replication. *Complementary Therapies in Medicine* 96 (4): 237–40, 1996.

Traditional Chinese Medicine

Beinfield, H., and E. Korngold. *Between Heaven and Earth: A Guide to Chinese Medicine.* New York: Ballantine, 1991.

————. Chinese traditional medicine: An introductory overview. *Alternative Therapies in Health and Medicine* 1 (1): 44–52, 1995.

Davis, S. The cosmological balance of the emotional and spiritual worlds: Phenomenological structuralism in traditional Chinese medical thought. *Culture, Medicine, and Psychiatry* 20: 83–123, 1996.

Kao, F. F. The impact of Chinese medicine on America. *American Journal of Chinese Medicine* 20 (1): 1–16, 1992.

Kaptchuk, T. *The Web That Has No Weaver: Understanding Chinese Medicine.* New York: Congdon and Weed, 1983.

Kubo, K., and H. Nanba. The effect of maitake mushrooms on liver and serum lipids. *Alternative Therapies in Health and Medicine* 2 (5): 62–66, 1996.

Wang, W. K., H. L. Chen, T. L. Hsu, and Y. Y. Wang. Alteration of pulse in human subjects by three Chinese herbs. *American Journal of Chinese Medicine* 22 (2): 197–203, 1994.

Journals

Alternative Therapies in Health and Medicine
Phone: (800) 345-8112
Fax: (610) 532-9001
www.healthonline.com/altther.htm

The American Journal of Natural Medicine
(800) 477-2995

Integrative Medicine
(520) 626-7222

Journal of Holistic Nursing
(520) 526-2196

Organizations/Associations

Acupuncture

American Academy of Medical Acupuncture
5820 Wiltshire Blvd, Suite 500
Los Angeles, CA 90036
Telephone: (213) 937-5514

American Association of Acupuncture and Oriental Medicine (AAAOM)
National Acupuncture Headquarters

1424 16th Street NW, Suite 501
Washington, DC 20036

National Acupuncture and Oriental Medicine Alliance
PO Box 77511
Seattle, WA 98177-0531
Telephone: (206) 524-3511
Fax: (206) 728-4841
E-mail: 76143.2061@compuserve.com

National Commission for the Certification of Acupuncturists
PO Box 97075
Washington, DC 20090-7075
Telephone: (202) 232-1404
Fax: (202) 462-6157

Ayurveda

Ayurvedic Institute
11311 Menaul NE, Suite A
Albuquerque, NM 87112
Telephone: (506) 291-9698

Billing codes

Alternative Link, LLC
1065 S. Main Street, Bldg C
Las Cruces, NM 88005
Telephone: (505) 527-0636
Web site: www.alternativelink.com

Chiropractic

American Chiropractic Association
1701 Clarendon Blvd
Arlington, VA 22209
Telephone: (703) 276-8800
Fax: (703) 243-2593
Web site: www.amerchiro.org/aca

Herbal Preparations

American Botanical Council
PO Box 201660
Austin, TX 78720
Telephone: (512) 331-8868

Herb Research Foundation
1007 Pearl Street, Suite 200
Boulder, CO 80302
Telephone: (800) 748-2617

Pharmacy Plus
JAG Group
629 Camino De Los Mares, Suite 304
San Clemente, CA 92673
Telephone: (714) 443-4010

Holistic Professional Associations

American Holistic Medical Association
4101 Lake Boone Trail, Suite 201
Raleigh, NC 27607
Telephone: (919) 787-5181

American Holistic Nurses' Association
PO Box 2130
Flagstaff, AZ 86003-2130
Telephone: (800) 278-AHNA
(520) 526-2196
Web site: www.ahna.org

Holistic Dental Association
PO Box 66609
Portland, NV 89102
Telephone: (702) 873-4542

Homeopathy

American Institute of Homeopathy
925 East 17th Avenue

Denver, CO 80218
Telephone: (303) 321-4105

International Foundation for Homeopathy
2366 Eastlake Avenue East, Suite 329
Seattle, WA 98102
Telephone: (206) 324-8230

National Center for Homeopathy
801 N. Fairfax Street, Suite 306
Alexandria, VA 22314
Telephone: (703) 548-7790
Fax: (703) 548-7792

Imagery

Academy for Guided Imagery
PO Box 2070
Mill Valley, CA 94942
Telephone: (800) 726-2070

Massage

American Massage Therapy Association
820 Davis Street, Suite 100
Evanston, IL 60201-4444
Telephone: (708) 864-0123
Fax: (708) 864-1178

Mind-Body Healing

Center for Mind-Body Medicine
5225 Connecticut Avenue NW, Suite 414
Washington, DC 20015
Telephone: (202) 966-7338
Fax: (202) 966-2589

Fetzer Institute
9292 West KL Avenue
Kalamazoo, MI 49009
Telephone: (616) 375-2000

Naturopathy

American Association of Naturopathic Physicians
2366 Eastlake Avenue East, Suite 322
Seattle, WA 98102
Telephone: (206) 328-8510
Fax: (206) 323-7612
Web site: infinity.dorsai.org/Naturopathic.Physician/

Bastyr University of Natural Health Sciences
College of Naturopathic Medicine
144 NE 54th
Seattle, WA 98105
Telephone: (206) 523-9585

Osteopathy

American Osteopathic Association
142 East Ontario Street
Chicago, IL 60611
Telephone: (312) 280-5882
(800) 621-1773, ext 7401

Reflexology

International Institute of Reflexology
PO Box 12462
St. Petersburg, FL 33733
Telephone: (813) 343-4811

Reflexology Research
PO Box 35820
Station D
Albuquerque, NM 87176
Telephone: (505) 344-9392
Fax: (505) 344-0246

Therapeutic Touch

Nurse Healers–Professional Associates International, Inc.
1211 Locust Street

Philadelphia, PA 19107
Telephone: (215) 545-8079

Trager Method

Trager Institute
33 Millwood Street
Mill Valley, CA 94941
Telephone: (415) 338-2688

Web Sites

Alternative Medicine Digest
www.alternativemedicine.com/alternativemedicine/

Alternative Therapies in Health and Medicine
E-mail: alttherapy@aol.com
www.healthonline.com/altther.htm

American Botanical Council
www.herbalgram.org/abcmission.html

American Herbal Pharmacopoeia
www.herbal-shp.org

Health World
206.135.37.254/clinic/therapy/herbal/index.html

Health World Online
www.healthy.net

The Herbal Bookworm
www/Teleport.com/janna/

HerbNet Magazine
www.herbalconnection.com

The Herb Research Foundation
www.herbs.org/herb/

Mariposa Botanicals
www.mariposabotanicals.com

Michael Moore's Home Page
www.rt66.com/hrbmoore/HOMEPAGE/HomePage.html

National Center for Homeopathy (NCH)
E-mail: nchinfo@igc.apc.org
Web site: www.healthy.net/nch

Office of Alternative Medicine,
National Institutes of Health
altmed.od.nih.gov/

Reflexology research
www.footweb.com/

Dr. Andrew Weil
www.drweil.com

APPENDIX B

Examples of Integrative Health Care Projects

This appendix provides examples of representative integrative healing projects. Projects developed as stand-alone efforts, as well as those that are components of larger health care systems, are included. Names of people to contact are provided when available; the actual person in the position may no longer be there, but the information can help reach the appropriate person or project.

University of Colorado Health Sciences Center, School of Nursing & Children's Hospital, Denver, CO

Project directors: Phyllis Updike, RN, DNS, School of Nursing;
Mary Jo Cleaveland, RN, MS, Children's Hospital;
Jan Nyberg, RN, PhD, School of Nursing
Contact: Dr. Updike; telephone: (303) 315-4315

The integration of complementary healing therapies into nursing practice for the care of children on the hematology-oncology-transplant unit of Children's Hospital, Denver, is a joint project between the School of Nursing and the Children's Hospital. The integration effort is designed as a program evaluation to examine the effectiveness of an educational program about complementary therapies on actual implementation in practice. The educational modules focus on integrative care and the specific complementary therapies of relaxation; guided imagery; massage; acupressure; Therapeutic Touch; and the use of music, sound, and silence. Also included is content related to spiritual dimensions and suffering in children and in those who care for them.

Pediatric Intensive Care Unit, UCLA Children's Hospital, Los Angeles, CA

Project directors: Nicholas G. Kasovac, MA, DTR, CMT,
Unit Service Coordinator III, PICU;
Clarice Marsh, RNC, NP, MS, Unit Director, PICU
Contact: Clarice Marsh; telephone: (310) 206-8149

This pilot program integrates dance/movement therapy, massage therapy, and Therapeutic Touch into the care of children in the pediatric intensive care unit. Parental involvement, trusting relationships, noninvasive touch, and examination of the effects of the program on children and their families are central components of the program.

University Center for Complementary and Alternative Medicine at Stony Brook, State University of New York, Stony Brook

Director: Samuel D. Benjamin, MD
Center telephone: (516) 444-3804

This center is supported by the second largest publicly funded research institution in the United States; it is a collaborative program that includes the Schools of Medicine, Nursing, Social Welfare, Health Technology and Policy Management, and Dentistry. The center is developing programs in service delivery, research, and education at both undergraduate and postgraduate levels. The program represents a health sciences, centerwide commitment to integrative health care that includes inpatient and primary care (both on- and off-site). The center offers acupuncture, herbal medicine, homeopathy, mind/body medicine, physical and manipulative medicine, spirituality, and subtle energies. It is exploring creative reimbursement options with managed care for both commercial and Medicaid products. SUNY will have at least one prospective outcome study with a managed care, Medicaid high-risk population, the first in the United States.

Arizona Center for Health and Medicine, Phoenix, AZ

Telephone: (602) 508-6800

This is an innovative group practice model that uses physicians, nurse practitioners, and physician's assistants as primary care providers. Alternative therapies integrated into care include acupuncture, homeopathy, Therapeutic Touch, guided imagery and relaxation, herbal preparations and nutritional supplements, therapeutic massage, the Trager method, the Feldenkrais method (bodywork), use of music and sound, and spirituality. The center is sponsored by Mercy Healthcare Arizona and Catholic Healthcare West. There is one large demonstration site and one smaller satellite site, both in the Phoenix metropolitan area. The main site's physical facilities were redesigned using architectural details, color, and art to reflect a healing environment in which to practice integrative health care.

Inova Heart Center, Inova Fairfax Hospital, Falls Church, VA

Contact: Mariece Huffman, CVOR Director; telephone: (703) 698-3166

This program is designed to instruct prospective cardiovascular surgical patients in the use of instrumental and voice-guided imagery tapes to reduce anxiety before, during, and after surgery. Patients receive a set of tapes several days preoperatively and are encouraged to listen to the tapes in the days prior to surgery to help them relax and then to bring the tapes with them when they go to the hospital for surgery. The tapes are used in the preoperative holding area and then again as patients awaken after surgery, in the intensive care and telemetry units. In addition, the cardiac catheterization laboratory and the coronary care unit have guided imagery tapes available for their patients as well.

In keeping with the integrative health care philosophy, the atmosphere in the cardiovascular operating room (CVOR) is designed to decrease patient anxiety. Prior to patients entering the CVOR, all sounds, including movement of equipment and instruments stops, and any music then playing ends as well. When patients enter, they hear only the music they have selected; the only other sounds are any necessary instructions being given by the anesthesiologist, nurses, or surgeons.

American Whole Health, Inc.

11150 Sunset Hills Road, Suite 210
Reston, VA 22090
Telephone: (703) 437-6336; *Fax:* (703) 437-1050

This company is a leader in providing integrative medicine in a for-profit group practice format. Currently it has three sites, but there are plans for more in various regions of the United States.

Columbia-Presbyterian Complementary Care Center

177 Fort Washington Avenue
New York, NY 10032
Telephone: (212) 305-9628
Directors: Mehmet Oz, MD, Co-founder/Executive Director; Jery Whitworth, RN, Co-founder/Director

This program has received much national press for its innovative program integrating alternative and complementary healing therapies, especially in the operating room experience. On admission, patients can elect to talk with an outreacher who explains integrative health care and helps them select from complementary therapies such as hypnosis, imagery, massage, and Therapeutic Touch. The program is designed for inpatients and is at the department level within the hospital system.

Center for Health and Medicine, St. Charles Medical Center, Bend, OR

Contact: Midge Cross, Program Director,
or Nancy Moore, RN, PhD, Vice President, Healing Health Services
Telephone: (541) 382-4321

The center's philosophic purpose is the creation of healthy lives through awareness and acknowledgment of the mind-body-spirit connection. Programs are designed to treat the whole person as well as the symptoms that patients may be experiencing. It is a component of St. Charles Medical Center, which is affiliated with the Healing Healthcare Project.

The center has a symptom reduction program, a Life Choice seminar, and a health coach service. It offers support and consultation to primary care practitioners who wish to integrate complementary healing therapies into their practice. The initial therapies being explored include acupuncture, Therapeutic Touch, Reiki (bodywork), guided imagery, tai chi, yoga, botanical medicine, mind/body medicine, neuromuscular therapy, osteopathic manipulation, and spirituality. The center is integrated with the hospital and physician practices to promote free flow of communication as the integrative effort proceeds.

Complementary Healing Services, Via Christi Regional Medical Center, Wichita, KS

Contact: Barbara Denison, RN, BSN, Director
Telephone: (316) 291-4325

The Department of Complementary Healing Services provides Therapeutic Touch, relaxation, imagery, massage, and music therapy to patients and staff in its facilities. Workshops for staff who want to learn Therapeutic Touch are provided as well. Community days are held for people who want to experience Therapeutic Touch from practitioners who have attended the workshops. Therapeutic Touch workshops and treatments, as well as educational sessions on stress management, are provided for staff, and treatments are provided for patients at no extra charge. Health care professionals can refer patients for these services or patients can self-refer.

Program in Integrative Medicine, The University of Arizona College of Medicine, Tucson, AZ

Director: Andrew Weil, MD, Program Developer
Telephone: (602) 626-7222

This program provides education and fellowship training for physicians who have completed a residency in family practice or internal medicine. Integration of a variety of alternative therapies into conventional care is emphasized. Students complete a two-year educational program that includes experience in integrative care at university-sponsored sites in Tucson. The center is a national site for postgraduate training and partners with other teaching institutions to develop integrative medical training programs.

University of Maryland School of Medicine, Center for Complementary Medicine, Baltimore, MD

Director: Brian Berman, MD
Telephone: (410) 448-6871

The center offers clinical services and emphasizes a strong research component, making it a national and international resource. It is one of the Office of Alternative Medicine research centers and specializes in evaluating complementary therapies for pain management.

Stanford Complementary Medicine Clinic

1101 Welch Road, Building A, Suite 6
Palo Alto, CA 94304
Director: David Spiegel, MD
Telephone: (650) 498-5566, *Fax:* (650) 498-5640

The focus of the clinic is on offering complementary medicine as an integrated component of conventional medical care. The program includes comprehensive evaluation and treatment planning, applied pyschophysiology and biofeedback, heart health support groups, hypnosis, medical acupuncture, mindfulness meditation, cancer support groups, therapeutic massage, and yoga.

Strang Cancer Prevention Center

428 East 72nd Street
New York, NY 10021
Director: Mitchell Gaynor, MD, Director, Medical Oncology and Integrative Medicine
Telephone: (212) 410-3820

Strang Clinic, where the PAP smear was developed, encourages integrative health care for cancer treatment and prevention. The clinic offers nutritional therapy, mind/body healing, guided imagery, music therapy, and herbal medicine.

John S. Marten Center for Complementary Medicine and Pain Management

St. Vincent's Hospital
8402 Harcourt Road, Suite 128
Indianapolis, IN 46260
Medical director: Wesley Wong, MD
Telephone: (317) 338-2536

This center integrates massage, acupuncture, biofeedback, guided visual imagery, yoga, meditation, and osteopathic manipulation for chronic pain management using a multidisciplinary approach.

Natural Health Clinic of Bastyr

1307 N. 45th Street
Seattle, WA 98103
Telephone: (203) 632-0354

Bastyr is the premier naturopathic medical college in the United States and has a Center of Excellence in HIV/AIDS research supported by the National Institutes of Health. The clinic integrates a full cadre of natural medical services. It is staffed by naturopathic physicians, acupuncturists, nutritionists, and psychologists. The AIDS clinic is staffed by allopathic physicians as well. The site delivers clinical services and serves as a teaching center for the university.

Community Health Centers of King County

403 East Meeker, Suite 300
Kent, WA 98031
Medical director: Martin Ross, MD
Telephone: (425) 277-1311

This is the country's first integrative community health center. The program integrates naturopathic physicians with allopathic physicians and other providers at one site.

INDEX

167